Severe Mental Illness in Primary Care

A companion guide for counsellors, psychotherapists and other professionals

Edited by
April Russello

Radcliffe Publishing
Oxford • New York

Radcliffe Publishing Ltd
18 Marcham Road
Abingdon
Oxon OX14 1AA
United Kingdom

www.radcliffe-oxford.com
Electronic catalogue and worldwide online ordering facility.

British Library Cataloguing in Publication Data

A catalogue record for this book is available from the British Library.

ISBN-13: 978 1 85775 765 1

Typeset by Ann Buchan (Typesetters), Middlesex
Printed and bound by TJI Digital, Padstow, Cornwall

Contents

Preface

This book was created with counsellors and psychotherapists in mind, as well as nurses and other primary care practitioners working in primary healthcare settings. The NHS and allied mental health systems can seem similar to a 'perpetual motion machine' due to the many changes that have continuously occurred over the past few years and even decades. Understanding this system can seem complex and puzzling even to staff who are working within the same system.

The wealth of information provided here about mental health and mental health systems could easily serve counsellors, psychotherapists and other practitioners as a 'companion guide' for those working in primary care, and who wish to understand how it all works. The information provided in this book is likely to be useful to practitioners, whether one has no knowledge of working in primary care, or is new to NHS work. However, for experienced NHS counsellors and other healthcare workers, this book can refresh and keep you thinking as well as maintaining your knowledge up to date.

It is likely, moreover, to be useful for all healthcare practitioners working in primary care because of its potential to encourage, incite, provoke, invite and elicit readers' (especially clinical practitioners') responses and thus reflection – reflection, on our own knowledge, conceptual positions, opinions and, hopefully, on our practice and knowledge as practitioners of the existing systems in primary care.

A wide variety of perspectives is provided – on the subjects of mental health, severe mental illness, dual diagnosis, counselling and mental health systems, mental illness and discrimination, mental illness and pain, how to find the evidence to research and much more. Some readers may find the information in this book totally new. Some may find it controversial – how can pain be an emotional response? Others may use it as a 'map' to help 'get one's bearings', when navigating through the NHS, and the concepts and information related to mental health, systems, mental health and pain and critical appraisal. Still others may find it refreshes what they already know and thus validates and confirms their sense of competence.

Each and every chapter offers the singular voice of the individual practitioner/ writer, conveying their individuality. The editor has made every effort to preserve 'the essence' of their meaning and message as they chose to express it. This book was not intended to be 'the definitive authority' on mental illness or severe and enduring mental illness. It has simply sought to offer readers some unique perspectives. These are offered by authors on their subjects of interest, often with passion, and certainly with expertise from their own personal knowledge. Each chapter in some way relates to, and invites the reader to explore, different perspectives and insights about mental health, mental health systems and, in one very different and important chapter, how we can become better researchers.

Ultimately, the individual and creative expression are what makes this book unique.

Robert John Ganderson (Chapter 1) privileges us with a first-hand account of an insider's journey through 'life after schizophrenia'. His is the book's 'Ordnance Survey map' whose story describes the landscape of mental illness and illustrates the truth and importance of 'belief in the hope of recovery' as described by Lester *et al* (2005). Robert John Ganderson is living proof that not every person with a severe and enduring mental health problem is, as the general stigma frequently attached to mental illness implies, a danger or a potential menace to society. Above all, we stand reminded that each, any and all of us, are entitled to a life, after a severe and enduring mental illness.

Hudson-Allez provides a pivotal 'foundation' chapter (Chapter 2) with descriptions of severe and enduring mental illnesses and their various presentations and considerations for assessment, as well as illustrating possible counselling treatments. She also identifies the distinctive role that counsellors can have in potentially informing and helping other staff, e.g. general practice receptionists, to refine their skills in identifying incoming patients with potential mental health problems.

My chapter (Chapter 3) attempts to describe the 'terrain' of mental health and to orient readers towards eliciting and recognising potential mental illness as well as speaking a 'common language'. Such a 'common language' does not mean that one subscribes to any particular 'theoretical' or 'medical' model, it is simply a way of communicating in a 'multidisciplinary mode' so that everyone will understand each other and work as a team to assist communication on how finally to best help the client/patient. The chapter invites readers to be aware of and possibly use existing mental health and wellbeing concepts and structures such as the 'three Ps' and the 'mental state examination' as systematic constructions that can potentially assist assessment and elicit possible mental ill-health and/or wellbeing.

Lester's chapter (Chapter 4) gives the reader a 'compass to the map'. It explains the seemingly 'mystical' workings of the NHS, the importance of mental health teams and how they work. The reader is invited to consider their own position in the 'coalface team' rather than be the 'outsider' counsellor, looking in.

Byng's chapter (Chapter 5) should be of great interest to counsellors, since it maps out potential models of care for individuals with severe and enduring mental health problems, including the innovative 'time banks' that build support from within communities themselves. Furthermore, in the 'Three Ds Model' there is much food for thought about who is included in this group.

Lipsedge's chapter on culture and mental illness (Chapter 6) exposes unhelpful attitudes that occur in relation to ethnic minorities. It invites readers to think about and reflect on interacting with clients who come from cultures, faiths and ethnic backgrounds that are different from our own. This chapter offers deep insight into the anguish and difficulties that are too frequently endured by such people who have a severe and enduring illness. The chapter also tries to clear up 'misunderstandings' that can occur when people work with those from different backgrounds, ethnicities and cultures. Crucially, however, it examines how these 'misunderstandings' can increase when the client or patient has a severe mental illness.

Freeth notes, with humour and wit, the use of acronyms and launches us into a very serious exploration of some of the politics around mental health (Chapter 7). This is a chapter that makes the reader want to 'do something', and it certainly makes one think. Although acronyms have been used in this book, this was solely due to space restrictions. The 'limited use' of such acronyms, as Rachel Freeth points out in her chapter, in mental health settings and for individuals with mental ill-health, are acknowledged with enthusiasm.

Harris (Chapter 8) reveals the interesting connection between physical and emotional pain. There appear to be common pathways and mechanisms in the development, appreciation and maintenance of emotional states such as anxiety and depression and the perception of pain. Readers of this chapter may be surprised, therefore, to learn about the close clinical correlation between pain syndromes and mental health phenomena.

Gerada gives a sombre account of the number of individuals with both substance abuse and mental health problems (Chapter 9). Certainly this chapter helps the reader to think about which one treats first. It highlights the necessity for as deep an understanding as possible of both serious mental illness and substance abuse and addiction when working with this group of people, and observes that the greater the complexity of the problem, the more the need for well-organised primary care.

It is unlikely that anyone would argue that there is a need for more counselling research; the research gaps in counselling and severe and enduring mental illnesses are bound to be generally wider since mental health is still not a 'required' element of most counselling qualification programmes (Eatock, 2004 and Chapter 11 of this book; Harris, 2004; Russello, 2004; Hudson-Allez, Chapter 2 of this book).

Curzio's chapter on critical appraisal (Chapter 10) guides readers into exactly how to seek and appraise mental health literature (or indeed all literature) they may need for an article, essay or presentation. This chapter offers counsellors an efficient route for how to commence an academic project in an accurate and effective manner that is relevant to high-quality research, an article or whatever the academic endpoint. What is more, it invites readers to consider forming clubs and groups to enhance critical thinking skills – so important in scholarship.

Finally Eatock offers an overview and summary (Chapter 11) of the chapters from his unique perspective as British Association for Counselling and Psychotherapy (BACP) Lead Adviser for Healthcare Counselling and Psychotherapy, and encourages us all to reflect on our practice with this particular group of individuals.

In brief, this combined work encourages the reader to reflect on mental health and mental ill-health and to perhaps challenge preconceptions. Readers are encouraged to think carefully about severe and enduring mental illness, and mental illness, and issues surrounding these topics. We are encouraged to consider whether individuals with such illnesses really are best served by limiting severe and enduring mental illness to diagnoses of a very specific set of particular illnesses such as the two recommended (schizophrenia and bipolar affective disorder) by the Sainsbury Centre (Cohen *et al*, 2004).

Finally, perhaps for many practitioners, it might be worth reflecting on, and perhaps questioning, the fact that most qualification counselling courses in the UK do not offer much, if any, training in mental health. This is despite the fact that, post-qualification, counsellors whether in private practice or the NHS or any other organisation, may, in all areas of employment, encounter individuals with mental health problems on their first day. With mental illness being 'one of the biggest causes of misery in our society' (Layard, 2004), are we really being well prepared?

April Russello
London, 2007

References

Cohen A, Singh SP and Hague J (2004) *The Primary Care Guide to Managing Severe Mental Illness.* London: The Sainsbury Centre for Mental Health Russell Press.

Eatock (2004) Editorial. *Healthcare Counselling and Psychotherapy Journal* 4(1):1.

Harris M (2004) GP Perspective. *Healthcare Counselling and Psychotherapy Journal* 4(1):20–1.

Layard R (2004) *Mental Health: Britain's biggest social problem?* Executive Summary London: Department of Health.

Lester H, Tritter JQ and Sorohan H (2005) Patients' and health professionals' views on primary care for people with serious mental illness; focus group study. *British Medical Journal* 330:1122.

Russello A (2004) SEMI trained or not? *Healthcare Counselling and Psychotherapy Journal* 4(1):2–5.

About the authors

Chapter 1: Robert John Ganderson's ambition to become a professional youth and community worker was shattered on being diagnosed with schizophrenia early in 1974. 'Down, but not out', he eventually managed to return to full-time employment, first in retailing, then as a customer service officer with a telecommunications company. Being made redundant in 1992 at the age of 48 he was again 'down, but not out'. He is now attempting to write a best-selling novel and hopes one day to join the ranks of Frederick Forsyth, Ruth Rendell and Jeffery Archer.

Chapter 2: Dr Glyn Hudson-Allez BSc(Hons) MSc(Forensic) PhD Dip. PST Dip Eat Dis Dip. Couns Dip. Ad Ed is a BPS chartered psychologist, specialising in counselling and forensic issues, and is a UK Counsellors and Psychotherapists (UKCP) registered psychosexual therapist. She has worked as a counsellor for 25 years, eight of which were in primary healthcare. She currently has a large private practice. She has published numerous papers, theses and book chapters, and two books: *Time Limited Therapy in a General Practice Setting* (London: Sage, 1997), and *Sex and Sexuality: questions and answers for counsellors and psychotherapists* (London: Whurr, 2005). She is currently writing her third book, about neuroscience and attachments. Glyn has a lifetime fellowship from the Association of Counsellors and Psychotherapists in Primary Care (CPC), and is former Training Manager for the British Association for Sexual & Relationship Therapy (BASRT).

Chapter 3: April Russello BFA MSc(mental health) Dip Couns BACP UKRC Reg PGCT in medical settings is a BACP accredited counsellor, has over 20 years' experience working in psychiatric and NHS general practice settings, and currently manages an East London counselling service in the NHS. She taught on the MSc in mental health at Kings College London from 1997 to 2003 and is currently engaged in PhD research studies at London South Bank University, Faculty of Health and Social Care.

Chapter 4: Dr Helen Lester MB Bch MA MD FRCGP is Professor of Primary Care at the University of Birmingham and has been a general practitioner (GP) in inner-city Birmingham for 15 years. She has a particular research and clinical interest in improving the primary care available for people with severe and enduring mental illness, particularly young people with first-episode psychosis.

Chapter 5: Dr Richard Byng MB Bch MRCGP MPH PhD is a GP who worked in Lewisham developing primary care mental health services. This included 'Mental Health Link', a programme to stimulate shared care for patients with long-term mental illness, and the development of the first health service-based 'time bank' in the UK. He is now a GP with a special interest in mental health in Plymouth PCT, and continues primary care mental health research at the Peninsula Medical School.

Chapter 6: Dr Maurice Lipsedge MPhil FRCP FRCPsych FFOM(Hon) has over 30 years experience of inner-city work. He is an Emeritus Consultant Psychiatrist at South London and Maudsley NHS Trust, and Visiting Senior Lecturer within Guys, Kings and St Thomas' School of Medicine. He has been widely referenced in the book he co-wrote with Roland Littlewood, *Aliens and Alienists: ethnic minorities and psychiatry* (1997) (3e, New York: Routledge). He also has numerous other publications, e.g. Mental health: access to care for black and ethnic minority people, in: Hopkins H and Bahl V (eds) (1993) *Access to Health Care for People from Black and Ethnic Minorities*. London: Royal College of Physicians, pp. 169–83; Religion and madness in history, in: Bhugra D (ed.) (1995) *Psychiatry and Religion*. New York: Routledge, pp. 23–50; Negotiating across culture, race and religion in the inner city, in: Okpaku S (ed.) (1998) *Clinical Methods in Transcultural Psychiatry*. Washington DC: American Psychiatric Association, co-written with Simon Dein.

Chapter 7: Dr Rachel Freeth BM DCP Dip Counselling is a general adult psychiatrist working for Gloucestershire Partnership NHS Trust. She gained a diploma in counselling (in the person-centred approach) in 1998 after taking a year out from psychiatry. Since then she has been particularly interested in bringing person-centred values and philosophy into psychiatric settings, writing about this in her book *Humanising Psychiatry and Mental Health Care. The challenge of the person-centred approach*. Oxford: Radcliffe Publishing, 2007.

Chapter 8: Dr Michael Harris MB ChB DA FRCA Dip Ph Med Dip MS Med qualified as a doctor in 1970, and as an anaesthetist in 1977. As well as continuing work in anaesthetics and general medicine, he has developed an interest in musculoskeletal medicine over the last 20 years, and obtained a special qualification in this field in 2000. The focus of his specialist work is now on the combination of pain management and orthopaedic medicine. He frequently encounters individuals presenting with patterns of pain that appear to have both a physical and psychological cause, and has become interested in the relationship between pain and mental ill-health.

Chapter 9: Dr Clare Gerada MBE FRCGP MRCPsych is a local GP in Lambeth, Project Director of the Royal College of General Practitioners (RCGP) Drugs Training Programme, and Director of Primary Care for the National Clinical Governance Support Team based in Leicester. She obtained the MBE in the 200th Birthday Honours for services in drug misuse and medicine. Her particular professional interest is improvement in drug misuse services within primary care at both local and national levels.

Chapter 10: Professor Joan Curzio PhD RGN is Director of Practice Development within the Faculty of Health and Social Care at London South Bank University. She is an experienced nurse who has been involved in research for over 20 years, with a focus in recent years on generic and specific ways of developing practice across a broad range of clinical areas including education developments, clinical role developments, and evaluation of new roles. She has published extensively and regularly presents on the topic of critical appraisal, which has included international audiences.

Chapter 11: The Revd John Eatock MA FBACP is Senior Counsellor with Bolton, Salford and Trafford NHS Mental Health Partnership, and Lead Adviser in Healthcare Counselling and Psychotherapy for the BACP. He is also Editor of the *Journal of Healthcare Counselling and Psychotherapy* and is particularly interested in counselling in general practice settings. His counsellor training was at the University of Manchester and the College of Ripon and York St John. John has written numerous articles in books and journals, been lecturer in counselling studies at the University of Salford and contributed to NHS documents and guidelines concerning mental health throughout the UK.

Abbreviations

AA	Alcoholics Anonymous
ACTT	assertive community treatment team
BACP	British Association for Counselling and Psychotherapy
BASRT	British Association for Sexual and Relationship Therapy
BMA	British Medical Association
BPD	borderline personality disorder
CBT	cognitive-behavioural therapy
CI	confidence interval
CMHT	community mental health team
CPA	care programme approach
CPC	Association of Counsellors and Psychotherapists in Primary Care
CPN	community psychiatric nurse
CRHTT	crisis resolution home treatment team
CSO	customer service officer
DSM	*Diagnostic and Statistical Manual of Mental Disorders*
DUP	duration of untreated psychosis
ECA	Epidemiological Catchments Area (Study)
EIS	early intervention services
FEP	first-episode psychosis
GMS	general medical services
GP	general practitioner
GPwSI	GP with a special interest
ICD	International Classification of Disease
ICP	integrated care pathway
LEDS	Life-Events and Difficulties Schedule
LTD	long-term depression
LTMI	long-term mental illness
MACA	Mental After Care Association
MSE	mental state examination
NICE	National Institute for Clinical Excellence
NSF	National Schizophrenia Fellowship/National Service Framework
OCD	obsessive–compulsive disorder
PCT	primary care trust

PHCT	primary healthcare team
PD	personality disorder
PTSD	post-traumatic stress disorder
QOF	Quality and Outcomes Framework
RCGP	Royal College of General Practitioners
RCT	randomised controlled trial
RMN	registered mental nurse
SEMI	severe and enduring mental illness
SIDDDs	safety, informal and formal care, diagnosis, disability and duration
SMR	standardised mortality rate
SSRI	Selective serotonin reuptake inhibitor
TENS	transcutaneous electrical nerve stimulation
UKCP	UK Counsellors and Psychotherapists
WRAP	wellness recovery action plan

Chapter 1

Living with chronic schizophrenia: is there life after schizophrenia?

Robert John Ganderson

In 1974, aged 30, I was diagnosed with chronic schizophrenia. It was a terrifying and traumatic experience, and my life changed dramatically as a result. Now, more than 30 years later, I have learned to live with this most debilitating illness, greatly aided by suitable and permanent medication. It has truly been a long and desperate struggle, during which I suffered one major relapse. Learning to live comfortably with my illness, however, has once again made my life purposeful and meaningful.

This is my story, which I shall detail in three sections: Before . . . Then . . . and Now.

Before

An only child, I was born on 7 July, 1944, in Newbury, Berkshire, where my mother was living with her sister and her four young children, away from our North London homes because of the war. My birth was a long and difficult one, but not unduly complicated. My father, exempt from military service on medical grounds, was an executive at the London head office of a company of retail wine merchants. He remained living in our flat above a company shop, in Winchmore Hill, throughout the war.

My paternal grandfather suffered a 'nervous breakdown' in the 1920s, as did two of my father's cousins and an uncle. My father's spinster sister spent three months in a local asylum in the 1930s, but managed to make a complete recovery. My father, although prone to occasional bouts of depression, remained free from mental illness all his life.

My mother, the youngest daughter of a doctor, had no history of mental illness on either side of her family. As a young girl she once witnessed the severe mental breakdown of an adult friend who was staying with my mother's family for a few days. This event upset her so much that for the rest of her life my mother refused to discuss the topic of mental illness, read articles about it, or watch any television programme concerning the subject; a cruel irony, therefore, that her son was to be diagnosed with schizophrenia. When this happened, my psychiatrist pleaded with her to visit me as frequently as possible, as I desperately needed both my parents' support in order to assist with some kind of a recovery – which, at the time, was considered doubtful. To my mother's immense credit she regularly visited me during my hospitalisation. Many years later she told me what a tremendous strain those visits were on her own mental health.

My mother was certainly aware of the series of 'nervous breakdowns' in my father's family, which she considered unfortunate, but insignificant. It was only later that my consultant psychiatrist told her, along with my father at a private meeting, that the 'breakdowns' concerned were most probably some form of schizophrenia, with a definite genetic link.

In the autumn of 1945 I returned to Winchmore Hill, and my aunt and cousins returned to their home in Edmonton, where my uncle was a doctor in general practice. I later attended a local Catholic primary school where I failed the eleven-plus exam yet managed to pass an entrance test to the collegiate all-boys' independent school conveniently located close to home.

I did not excel in the classroom or on the playing field, and because of numerous (physical) illnesses in my early years at this school I was invariably in the bottom five of the class in examinations. I was a fluent reader but a slow learner, and suffered a degree of bullying as a result. The teachers, with the exception of a geography master from New Zealand, generally regarded me as incorrigible, and with negligible prospects of achieving any academic qualifications. Reluctantly, my parents allowed me to leave the collegiate, aged 17, without sitting any GCE examinations.

That year (1961) I soon found a job as a junior salesman in a family-owned retail sports business, comprising three shops in North London. Being interested in self-defence, I joined a local judo club. Having had something of an aggressive temperament in my boyhood and youth, I was well suited to my new sport. With enthusiasm and perseverance I managed to attain first Dan, black belt status, within seven years.

By 1970, aged 26 and still living at home with my parents, I had been promoted to branch manager of one of the sports shops, and had co-founded a thriving judo club in Winchmore Hill, where I was now spending most of my free time. I was suddenly very unhappy, however, because of a break-up in my first serious relationship. This was with a girl I had met through judo; we were very much in love, but she was not content with dating me on an occasional basis. Another problem at this time was that my mother was becoming unbearably possessive with me; this had such a disturbing effect that I decided to start a new life for myself in another country – New Zealand.

Officials at New Zealand House in London were dismissive about my prospects of emigration, telling me that only trades-people and those from acknowledged professions were eligible for government subsidy. At that time, British citizens could easily enter New Zealand without visas, but travelling there was very expensive.

Having no relations or friends in New Zealand, I concluded that it made sense to find a job there prior to leaving the UK. Deciding that '*I can and I will*', I placed an advertisement in three independent New Zealand publications:

EXPERIENCED SPORTS RETAIL MANAGER (26) COMING TO NEW ZEALAND, SEEKS SUITABLE EMPLOYMENT (Contact details)

Thinking that the chances of a response were practically nil, I concentrated on saving as much money as possible in order to finance my intended migration.

Incredibly, a director of a large and well-established sporting business, recovering in an Auckland hospital from a minor operation, read my advertisement and sent me a job application form.

Consequently, I was offered, and accepted, a position as a senior salesman in their Auckland store. Amazingly, I also qualified for a government subsidy for my air fare, by way of a newly introduced scheme for British citizens accepted for employment by reputable New Zealand businesses. The long and complex formalities eventually completed, I departed from Heathrow for Auckland on 27 October 1970.

Residing at the local YMCA, I enjoyed life and work in Auckland for approximately eight months. Then, somewhat unsettled, and with my employer's agreement, I left and flew to Brisbane, Australia, with a YMCA friend who was returning home to Cairns.

After a few days of sightseeing, I flew to Darwin where, I had been assured, highly paid labouring work was plentiful. This proved not to be the case but, confident that 'where there is a will, there is a way', I managed to find a job as a civilian storeman at the local Army barracks. Unable to tolerate the intense heat, however, I left after seven weeks, by coach, for Alice Springs and from there to Perth, Western Australia, by train.

Residing at the city YMCA I also managed to gain employment there as an assistant youth worker and judo instructor. A few weeks later the YMCA hostel manager, by way of a friend of his, found me a job as a canteen manager at Useless Loop, an outback mining camp. This was an intensely stressful and hellish experience.

Working shift hours, seven days a week, I was highly paid, but the stresses of the work concerned, physically and mentally, resulted in my quitting and returning to Perth within three months.

I then journeyed, via Adelaide, by train, to Melbourne, where I found myself a job as a storeman in a large grocery and confectionery warehouse. I lodged in the city YMCA, and spent eight enjoyable months there before deciding to move to Sydney.

Taken on at the Sydney warehouse of my former employer, I lodged at a guest house in a local suburb for the next 16 months. I then decided that it was time to return home for a visit (September 1973), and my boss granted me eight weeks' unpaid leave to do this.

Overjoyed at being home again, however, I decided to apply for work as a full-time youth leader. Failing to gain admittance to the YMCA training college, but remembering that 'there is always a way' to do what you really want to do, I was accepted as a full-time leader at the Harrow Youth Club in Hammersmith, which is owned by Harrow School.

There I worked on a shift basis for five and sometimes six days a week, and was studying hard for a formal qualification for my newly chosen career. Everything went well at first, but somewhat inevitably, the increasing mental stress of coping with rowdy and ill-disciplined teenagers, combined with long night hours of academic study, and increasingly less and less sleep, began to take their toll on my mental health.

Then

One Friday evening, early in May 1974, having just left the Harrow Club, exhausted and agitated, a voice suddenly screamed out in my head 'the man behind you is going to kill you'.

Panicking, I turned round and stared into the eyes of a man several paces behind me. He stopped and stared back, so I ran as fast as I could into Hammersmith Underground station, only slightly relieved to find that the would-be assassin was nowhere in sight.

Then the 'voice' told me that the man knew where I lived, and that he was going to come and kill me sometime that evening. Intensely nervous, all the way home I kept looking out for him, convinced that he was somewhere in the shadows behind me. At home, my parents quickly realised that I was in a deep state of psychosis. I tried to persuade my father to telephone the police and summon an officer to patrol outside the flat throughout the night.

Somehow, he managed to calm me down assuring me that he would call the police provided I went straight to bed. He emphasised that I was quite safe at home, with all windows and doors locked. However, I passed most of the night endlessly walking round my bedroom, arguing with the demon voice as it continually taunted me about my impending death. Eventually, I collapsed on the bed and fell into a troubled sleep.

Early the next morning I was awakened by a series of loud banging noises somewhere out in the street. Immediately, a 'voice' told me that these noises were made by two men with cylinders of poison gas which they were going to use to kill me.

All my energy drained from me and I began, between floods of tears, crying out for help. My parents persuaded me to come with them, by the back door – so as to avoid the two men – to see my uncle, my doctor, who they repeatedly assured me would quickly help me to get better. On the way there, by car, another 'voice' told me that I had incurable bowel cancer.

My uncle saw me in his surgery, which adjoined the house, and I told him that I had bowel cancer, saying nothing about the troublesome voices, convinced that if I did mention them he would immediately give me a lethal injection.

Having given me an internal examination he assured me that I did not have bowel cancer, but said that he would like me to go to hospital for a further examination by another doctor. He then told me to wait while he went back into the house to telephone the North Middlesex Hospital. Unbeknown to me, of course, he was arranging for my emergency admittance to their psychiatric unit.

My mother drove me there while my father kept assuring me that I would soon be much better. My uncle also drove to the hospital as he knew the consultant psychiatrist quite well; the consultant being off duty, however, my uncle arranged admission formalities with another psychiatrist, and I was allocated a bed and heavily sedated.

I remained an inpatient for seven weeks, during which I was given numerous different drugs – lithium and Largactil are two that I remember – before being prescribed one that I responded favourably to: Stelazine. At first, however, initial heavy doses resulted in giving me a disturbing side-effect: fits of involuntary shaking. This was eased somewhat by my being given yet another drug – Artane . . . I would describe the effects of such doses of medication as like trying to breathe while walking under the sea. That's how it felt to me . . . I think many similar patients are still heavily medicated to this day.

During those early weeks I tried to wander from the ward several times, and was duly escorted back by a nurse or two; on one occasion, apparently, it took the combined efforts of three male nurses to do this because I suddenly became aggressive. Recounting this event, embarrassingly, many years later to an old judo friend, he responded with a laugh '*only* three? With your judo grade it should have taken six at least!' Humour did have, and still has, a therapeutic effect on me and others too, I suspect.

The voices in my head became less frequent as the weeks went by, but one evening while watching the ward television, the programme host – Hughie Green – suddenly began to talk to me personally, saying that he would like me to appear on his show. This caused me to panic, resulting in an emergency visit from the duty doctor and an immediate dose of a powerful sedative.

In addition to being treated with drugs I also had to attend occupational therapy classes each weekday morning from 10 am to 12 noon in a large workshop in an annex to the main hospital building. Here we could choose to do art (painting); woodwork; needlework; printing, or mosaic work. Choosing to do mosaic work I duly made several ashtrays, among other items, which I was allowed to keep. Although heavily medicated, I found this practical occupation helpful.

In the afternoons, there were occasional group-therapy sessions for me to attend, comprising between eight and twelve patients and a psychiatrist. These I personally found to be interesting and helpful, enabling me to retain a semblance of social interaction; but there were mixed reactions from other attending patients. I recall one occasion when a female patient started screaming loudly and became hysterical on being asked to talk, inappropriately, I with hindsight felt, about an upsetting incident in her childhood. The therapist had persuasively pressed the incident from her, but the next day she attempted suicide.

I was fortunate that my psychiatrist understood and explained to my parents the importance of support, and they duly visited me every day. This was undoubtedly a distressing experience for them, especially so for my mother whom I remember crying on most of these occasions. After five weeks of confinement to the ward, and responding well to Stelazine, my dosage was reduced, and I was allowed home at weekends – from Friday afternoon to early Sunday evening. After two such weekends I was discharged, thereafter attending as a day patient for five days a week for the following five weeks.

I was then required to visit a psychiatrist in the outpatients clinic, once every three months for three years.

Early in September 1974, my father drew my attention to an advertisement in the local paper for an assistant manager at the sports shop where I was formerly employed as a manager. I successfully applied for this post and happily returned to a comfortable work environment, serving many customers whom I had got to know well in earlier years.

Now on a new medication which greatly suited me – Triptafen tablets – I gradually made an excellent recovery. Socially I became active again: teaching occasional self-defence courses for scout troops and youth clubs; infrequently going out in the company of old friends; occasionally going on my own to a theatre or cinema.

In 1978, a friend who worked for a large telecommunications organisation suggested I apply there for a storeman's job that he knew was vacant. I applied and obtained that job. Again, I was fortunate to have a friend to recommend me.

During my obligatory medical examination I mentioned that I had suffered a nervous breakdown four years ago, and emphasised that I had made a complete recovery. This was accepted without question, probably because (1) the nature of the warehouse work is mundane and relatively stress free, and (2) my employment record was a good one. I then passed an assessment interview and although I was offered a more difficult storeman's post, I accepted an easier clerical post.

Employment was and still can be, I believe, a tremendous difficulty for individuals diagnosed with schizophrenia or other mental health problems, not only because of potential stress on the individual but also because of the significant stigma attached to having a mental health problem.

I started there in the first week of February 1979 and quickly settled into a relatively easy work schedule, with a most agreeable team of colleagues and management.

When my father died from prostate cancer in January 1980, my uncle advised me to take an extra Triptafen tablet at night for the next few weeks, thus enabling me to mentally cope with the bereavement. In June 1982, my boss asked me to formally apply for a newly created post within the company. As a customer service officer (CSO), I worked with the public answering fault reports, diagnosing faults, and allocating them to appropriate engineers.

I passed the interview, then a two-week mandatory engineering course, and soon settled down in my new work, together with five female CSOs, operators and new, like myself, to engineering work.

In my late 30s, I happily established a steady relationship with a divorced lady, two years my junior, whom I had met at a local cheese and wine evening. Triptafen must not be mixed with alcohol, but I was allowed the occasional evening free from my medication to enjoy a glass or two of wine, or a pint of beer. Jane (not her real name) had a cousin who suffered with schizophrenia, and I could comfortably discuss this illness with her. Our relationship blossomed to the extent that we were discussing marriage. Then, in June 1984, Jane was diagnosed with advanced ovarian cancer, and died barely three months later. Intensely distraught, I stopped taking my medication, slept very little, and began drinking quite heavily in the evenings and at weekends to try and relieve my grief; it didn't work. For a few weeks everything went quite well, and I convinced myself that I now no longer needed my medication.

Then, quite suddenly, again, I began hearing voices while talking to a customer who was reporting a fault. There were two voices in conversation this time, both discussing my imminent death. I terminated the call and burst into tears telling my boss that I was not well, but not mentioning the voices in my head. He and my colleagues were very sympathetic and an engineer took me home in his car.

My mother was out when I arrived home: suddenly, another voice told me that when the cuckoo clock struck 13 times it was going to blow up and kill me; it was now just before noon. Panicking, I telephoned my work headquarters and told my colleague who answered that I was going to die soon, and that I especially wanted her and all my other colleagues to come to my funeral; I then slammed the receiver down.

Shortly afterwards my mother returned, realised that I needed help and begged me to let her telephone my new doctor (my uncle had recently retired) who, coincidently, she worked for as a receptionist. Angrily, I grabbed her at the throat with both hands; bursting into tears she cried out 'whatever you do to me I will still love you'. The cuckoo clock struck thirteen and I ran screaming into my bedroom and collapsed on the bed.

My mother telephoned my doctor, who instructed her to give me three Triptafen tablets immediately, and telephone him early the next morning if I was still very disturbed. Somehow, I took the tablets and managed some tormented sleep, but was woken in the early hours by another voice in my head taunting me once again about my imminent death.

My doctor duly arrived, called an ambulance, and I was taken to the psychiatric ward of Chase Farm Hospital, Enfield, where I was immediately admitted to a room adjoining a ward, and heavily sedated.

I do not remember much about the next few days, except that on one occasion I ran naked from my room into the main ward screaming at the top of my voice about a 'voice' tormenting me. I vaguely remember being restrained by two female nurses, returned to my room and sedated.

Surprisingly, I quickly and positively responded to heavy doses of amitriptyline and was discharged within two weeks. The consultant psychiatrist emphasised in our final private meeting at the hospital, that I must continue taking Triptafen tablets for the rest of my life. Following another two weeks of convalescence at home, I was able to return to work, where I was welcomed back.

Slowly but surely my life began to return to some kind of normality, although I remained heartbroken at the loss of one whom I loved so much, and who had been so involved with my future.

Largely to combat my grief, but also to improve my education, I purchased, and successfully completed, correspondence courses in English, creative writing, and sales and marketing. As a result, I gained a few acknowledged qualifications including the Licentiateship in Sales and Marketing from the City and Guilds of London (equivalent to an NVQ level four).

In 1990, my company headquarters moved to another location where, two years later, a massive company reorganisation resulted in my accepting a lucrative redundancy deal. My elderly mother moved from our rented flat into sheltered accommodation and I moved to a guest house in Galway, Southern Ireland – a favourite annual holiday haunt over many years.

Unable to find suitable employment, however, I returned to London six months later, where a chance encounter with an old friend resulted in my moving into his holiday flat in Sussex, where I stayed for the next eight months. Unsettled and reaching the age of 50 in July 1994, I decided to return to London.

Before doing so I telephoned the National Schizophrenia Fellowship (NSF), now Rethink, requesting guidance concerning suitable accommodation in Greater London. They promptly sent me a three-page list of housing associations catering for people with mental health problems. This organisation is an excellent support for people with schizophrenia who are trying to help themselves.

From this list, I randomly chose the Carr-Gomm Society Ltd, a national and charitable housing association, and well represented in London. My interview was successful and my name was entered onto their waiting list. I soon moved into private lodgings in North London to be nearer to my mother, and closer to London in readiness for another move. In April 1995, I moved into a Carr-Gomm house in Islington where a support worker catered for seven single people, each with their own room, but who shared communal facilities. Qualifying for income support (now jobseeker's allowance), I also began the difficult task of seeking employment: difficult because of my age and ageism. I had also been advised by two independent psychiatrists to disclose to any prospective employer, the fact that I suffered with schizophrenia. This disclosure policy often meant my being vulnerable to the stigma potential employers attach to this illness.

Further medical advice also meant that I must avoid any kind of work that involved any degree of mental stress. The disability adviser at the local job centre was both sympathetic and helpful, but although I managed to obtain a few interviews – mostly with retailers – no job offers resulted. I did hold a full driving licence, but was precluded from making use of it because of the 'drowsiness' side-effect of my permanent medication.

I was spending most of the week in Islington, and weekends with my mother who, in spite of her advanced years, was still able to manage her small home and personal affairs. In June 1996, I accepted an offer from Carr-Gomm to move into a small independent flat, one of six in a large North London house, recently purchased and converted by the society.

Financially, this was something of a struggle because, although housing benefit were paying my rent and council tax, I was responsible for all household bills – now invoiced to me personally. Then came a serious blow to my physical health – I suddenly began to suffer infrequent spasms of severe back pain, subsequently being diagnosed with spinal arthritis and chronic spondylitis.

This resulted in my suffering acute bouts of depression, but then two things happened that considerably improved my personal circumstances.

Firstly, a jobseeker adviser suggested that I ask my doctor to certify me as needing income support for both mental and physical reasons. This he did, and some months later I was granted permanent sickness benefit, at a much higher rate than jobseeker's allowance. Not having to worry any longer about finances was indeed a burden lifted from my shoulders.

Secondly, I began a meaningful relationship with my immediate neighbour in our Carr-Gomm Home. Carolyn is 20 years younger than me and physically disabled; when barely six months old, she became very ill with meningitis, which left her semi-paralysed in her left leg, and with limited use of a deformed left hand.

In spite of the inevitable problems of her disability, Carolyn is always cheerful, uncomplaining, and very much an inspiration to me. We may be years apart in age, but we share a common interest in many things including pop music, reading, and enjoying local walks.

As the year 2000 approached, my life began to blossom once again, with the promise of living comfortably and securely in medical retirement – and completely at ease, at long last, with a distressing mental illness. Having someone to share my life with, who means so much to me, is the biggest blessing of all however. Relationships are important for most people, and perhaps especially for people with mental health problems, who may experience long bouts of isolation.

Now

Personally, one sad and traumatic event that occurred on 4 December in the year

2000 was the death of my mother, aged 89 years. Physically frail and increasingly confused mentally, she had moved into a local care home in September that year, where she had settled in quite well. I regularly visited her and, happily, she always recognised and welcomed me.

I was deeply distressed at her passing but thanks to Carolyn, bless her, I managed to organise and attend her funeral, with much sadness but only a minimum of mental stress. My mother had stood by me stoically when I was so ill mentally. She had visited me every day when I was admitted to Chase Farm Hospital, and greatly assisted with my convalescence afterwards, in spite of her lifelong (and personally distressing) possessiveness of me. I will, nevertheless, eternally remember her with great love and immense gratitude.

Since 1996 I have been an active member of Rethink (formerly the NSF), taking every opportunity to increase my knowledge and understanding about schizophrenia, and the progress being made by way of new drugs and treatment programmes. I infrequently attend a number of their functions each year, and am registered with them as a media volunteer. A group of approximately 200 service users, we are 'on call' to talk about our individual experiences of mental illness with journalists from local and national publications, as well as those representing radio and television.

We meet occasionally, usually in London, in a relaxed and informal atmosphere, and discuss matters of common interest. At our last meeting we were joined by two journalists from different publications, the main topic being the media's role in combating the stigma of mental illness. It was a lively and positive debate, and everyone agreed that the event was a huge success. Being involved in helping others who have suffered as I did has given me enormous personal satisfaction.

Rethink's quarterly magazine *Your Voice* is interesting, topical, and informative. The organisation also campaigns, publicly and politically, on a variety of issues relevant to those suffering with mental illness, for example, alerting the public, especially teenagers, to the dangers of smoking cannabis. It should perhaps be mentioned at this point that I personally have never experimented with any kind of illegal drug or substance.

One Rethink campaign of personal interest is that of the 'forgotten generation'; this refers to a large group of people with mental illness living in society, largely forgotten by mainstream health services. For the most part these are people who have lived with a severe mental illness for many years. They now live their lives without the all-round help and support that would allow them to raise their quality of life.

It is a sad fact that in terms of mental health reforms, this group of people seems to have been forgotten – bearing in mind that I could have become one of these people, but for my strong sense of 'where there's a will . . .' and my family medical connections.

In terms of treatment for schizophrenia, it is pleasing to note that there are many more drugs available now than when I was first diagnosed with this illness, back in 1974. However, a large number of these have distressing side-effects that invariably cause additional and complex problems for the recipient – physical and psychological, sometimes both.

I feel strongly, therefore, that psychiatrists and their staff teams should very carefully assess the use of such drugs on a case-by-case basis. Evidence of side-effect problems is widespread; *Your Voice* infrequently details disturbing cases of patients/service users suffering horrendous side-effects, sometimes with truly devastating consequences, having been prescribed certain psychotic drugs.

These side-effects differ, from frequent cases of chronic obesity, blunted or reduced emotional responsiveness, to occasional incidents of liver damage. Additionally, of course, some physical side-effects also seem to incur various psychological problems that also need to be dealt with.

Without doubt, the most frightening and troubling aspect of schizophrenia is hearing voices. Sadly, as I am reliably informed, there is no drug as yet that will eliminate this most disturbing condition. However, progress is being made in this direction and, given time, future drugs will ideally have only a minimum of 'tolerable' side-effects, as well as 'hopefully' minimising those demon voices – thus enabling a swift recovery back to normality.

In my own case history, it has to be admitted that I have been fortunate in ways that many other adult sufferers of schizophrenia have not: I quickly responded to, and became stable with, a drug having only a minimum of side-effects; I was able to quickly return to a comfortable work environment after being discharged from hospital, on two occasions; I managed to sustain a steady employment record from 1974 until 1992; and I now regularly receive a low, but adequate, level of support via Carr-Gomm staff.

Even at 61 years of age, and 'medically retired' when my general practitioner (GP) signed me off, I still keep busy and active in order to keep fit – mentally as well as physically. Apart from my involvement with Rethink, I am currently working on three independent correspondence courses – no pressure here, as there are no set deadlines to meet – and am also attempting to write a novel!

Yes, thankfully, I am a survivor of a terrible mental illness but, medication aside, my own important personal contribution has been to work very hard in order to reach the stability and peace of mind that I now value so highly.

In summary: with energy, determination and persistence I have pursued a simple philosophy . . . 'I can and I will; where there is a will, there is a way; and there is always a way'.

So, yes, there is life after schizophrenia.

Chapter 2

Counselling individuals with severe and enduring mental illness

Glyn Hudson-Allez

Introduction

Severe and enduring mental illness (SEMI), as Russello (2004) has outlined, is a term that describes a constellation of disorders that are chronic and persistent over time and lead to moderate to high enduring dysfunction and disability. Following the fairly recent shift from hospital-based 'institutional' care to community-based 'social care' programmes, many individuals with SEMI find themselves living within the community, and therefore by default, have more interaction with primary care services than secondary care. Indeed, Kendrick (2004) points out that 25–30% of patients with SEMI lose contact with the secondary services and are entirely looked after within primary care. These individuals may also experience co-morbid conditions; as Gerada points out in her chapter on dual diagnosis later in this book (*see* Chapter 9), these individuals may also have concomitant substance addiction, and co-morbid conditions like depression or anxiety, and may well have additional reactions to negative life events. Thus they too will be bereft from grief, traumatised by victimisation, or suffer the pain or loss of relationship breakdown, and may therefore be referred to the primary care counsellor for help.

The majority of counselling training, however, offers little or no information on dealing with a person with a mental illness, let alone the skills training required to work with the enduring difficulties like disturbance of thought processes. This chapter will discuss an approach to counselling people with SEMIs, by careful assessment of the presenting issues. It will briefly look at various models, including person-centred, psychodynamic and cognitive-behavioural approaches, and then move on to the presenting symptoms and their related issues that can be the focus of the counselling work.

Mental health presentation

Mental health and illness 'presentations' can vary between individuals, across populations, and even within the same diagnostic category. Increasingly, our understanding of mental health is on a spectrum of presentations, where individuals move along a continuum of severity in different phases of their lives, or in different cycles of their illness (Bentall, 2003). This means that the traditional categorical classification of presentation becomes somewhat less useful in clinical work, as many people do not always fit into the neat descriptions of the *Diagnostic and Statistical Manual of Mental Disorder* (DSM IV). It is essential, therefore, that counsellors have a thorough knowledge of mental health and illness presentation as part of their basic training, as well as having an understanding of the variability of presentation, so that their assessment, formulations and interventions are based on knowledge and the clinical literature.

As presentations of SEMIs are complex and multifaceted, sometimes the counsellor may experience uncertainty as to whether some of the more 'unusual' presentations are open to counselling interventions. Maher (1988), however, proposed that delusions and hallucinations serve a function within a psychosis, as a reasonable attempt to defend against the possibility of going mad. It is important, therefore, to acknowledge that some people who have what may be described as psychotic experiences, may not have contact with mental health services at all, because they do not find their hallucinations distressing. Indeed, 10–15% of the population have heard voices or experienced hallucinations at some time in their lives (Tien, 1991), and have developed strategies for living with them. The only difference between the two populations of those who sought help and those who coped were that the latter felt they were stronger than their voices, whereas the former thought they were weaker.

A study by Bak *et al* (2005) has emphasised this distinction by finding that childhood trauma predisposes people to suffer more emotional distress in the face of psychotic experiences, than those who had no traumatic history. This study offers an explanation for the association of the incidence of sexual, emotional and physical abuse experienced in the childhood histories of those individuals with schizophrenia. Indeed, Read *et al* (2004) reviewed 13 studies of schizophrenic populations and found that the incidence of trauma in the histories of these individuals ranged from 51% to 97%. And from the discipline of neuroscience, there has been compelling evidence of permanent changes to the hippocampal-limbic areas of the brain as a result of severe abuse and neglect (Teicher, 2002) with consequential psychiatric presentations (Kendler *et al*, 2000). In addition, as Read (2005) has argued, poverty, urban living, discrimination, and having a battered mother in childhood have all been shown to be predictive of adult psychosis.

Fowler *et al* (1995) proposed the vulnerability-stress model, which offers a formulation of schizophrenia that, while recognising biological influences on psychosis, also focuses on the way that behaviour, beliefs and experiences shape a psychotic illness. This model provides a basis for counselling interventions that also provide information-giving and skilled-based strategies to enhance the client's social functioning.

Mental health team working

Counsellors working in primary care need to consider themselves as working as part of the primary healthcare team, and as such are not working with this client group alone. In addition to the counsellor, the team will consist of the GP, who has primary clinical responsibility for the patient, practice and district nurses, health visitors, and, in some of the larger practices, social workers and psychologists. Some GPs have undertaken specific specialist training in mental health and psychiatry, whereas others may have little understanding, interest or knowledge of mental or psychological health. Team and practice meetings can therefore be vital as a means of sharing knowledge and experience with each other, and building up trust in collaboration of who is the best team member to provide which part of the treatment to the patient. Because of the diversity of clinical experience in mental health, team meetings will also build up a shared language about presenting mental health issues, so that all members are clear as to what might be considered a minor transient distress as opposed to the precipitation of a major psychotic episode which is often, but not always, an acute problem needing clear and rapid intervention. Unfortunately, too often counsellors have kept themselves aloof from practice meetings, fearing that their confidentiality ethic might be compromised, and as a consequence, a vital learning opportunity within the team is lost.

Shared knowledge about the patient and the family history also varies within the team, and receptionists are often a valuable resource of family information, which can be vital in terms of understanding each individual's presentation. Receptionists are the first port of call for patients, and often patients may share information with them that they do not share with the GP. Counsellors should be encouraged to talk with receptionists regarding people with a SEMI and perhaps, if relevant, offer guidance as to how to recognise mental ill-health and the best way for such patients to be dealt with on arrival at reception. For example, a patient with paranoia may have a real difficulty with sitting in the waiting room with other patients, or alternatively other patients may respond in a negative way to a patient behaving in an unusual manner. Additional family information may enhance the decision-making process if it is thought that the secondary care services need to be involved for the patient to receive additional support in the absence of a family support network.

Good links with the secondary care services or community mental health team (CMHT) are also of great importance for counsellors in primary care. This team may comprise psychiatrists, clinical and counselling psychologists, psychotherapists, occupational therapists, social workers, and community psychiatric nurses (CPNs), and can offer valuable support, assessments of patients, and advice to the GP regarding appropriate prescribing for the patients. It is a very fortunate team, however, that has all of these professionals to hand for collaborative work. There may also be counsellors who work in secondary care in some areas of the country. Where good links are built up with members of the secondary services, these can be valuable assets for the counsellor and the general practice, to be able to seek advice regarding concerns about a particular client presentation.

Under the National Institute for Clinical Excellence (NICE) (2002) guidelines, the GP is required to place the patient's name on a register to monitor his or her situation, and make sure that the patient receives routine check-ups for their physical wellbeing as well as ensuring they are maintaining their psychotropic medication. However, research has suggested that SEMI registers in different practices have varying outcomes in terms of the benefits for the individual and their contact with the mental health services (Barr, 2000). In the first national survey of mental health in primary care (Mental After Care Association (MACA), 1999), it was found that only 13% of GPs had had any experience of mental health training in the previous 5 years, yet they considered that it accounted for 30% of their workload. This seems to suggest that the GP may be very open to mutual support from the primary care counsellor in dealing with patients presenting with SEMI.

Counselling assessment

The severity of a person's illness may not be readily obvious at the outset, thus the counsellor's approach to a client with SEMI may well be influenced by the amount of information received beforehand, either via the referral letter, or verbally from a colleague who may have encountered the individual before. Sometimes, preconceptions can hinder the valuable work that can be achieved. However, there are some important aspects that the counsellor needs to consider before embarking on a counselling contract. Box 2.1 shows the usual considerations of assessment, especially if the counsellor is working on a short-term contract.

Box 2.1   Assessment considerations

- What problems is the person experiencing?
- What would he or she like to change?
- What is their view of why this is happening now?
- Are there any life events or stressors?
- What support networks are in place?
- What is their life history; is there a history of trauma and/or abuse?
- What are their skills, abilities and coping strategies?
- What is their level of self-esteem?
- What is their attachment style – could they cope with the loss of the counselling relationship in 6/12 sessions?
- What medication are they taking and what is their level of compliance with this? What effect is this having in terms of functioning and side-effects?
- Is there an issue with alcohol or drugs? (Studies suggest that substance misuse occurs in 30–50% of this population (George, 2004).)
- Is there is a risk of personal neglect, self-harm or harm to others?
- What help is he/she receiving from other services?
- What has helped in the past?
- What additional help or support does he/she need now?

There are potentially similar assessment questions that might be considered in any other potential counselling contract, although of course not all professionals would necessarily be interested in 'attachment styles' or in conducting this exact form of assessment. However, in the case of a person with a SEMI, the counsellor may find that other healthcare professionals are monitoring the individual more closely. For example, the GP is also required to assess drug compliance, as an unwillingness to take medication may lead to a return of symptoms such as hearing voices, and eventually enforced hospitalisation. This takes the aspect of control and individual rights away from the person, which may be an issue raised in the counselling room.

Risk assessment

The aim of risk assessment is to promote safety for the client and the counsellor (and sometimes significant others), inform care planning and act as a guide to the therapeutic encounter, enabling the counselling work to be done. Although risk assessment is an everyday aspect of counselling, a more thorough risk assessment needs to be undertaken with individuals with a SEMI. Assessment of the person's mental health issues may already have occurred on the basis of SIDDDs: safety, informal and formal care, diagnosis, disability and duration (Slade *et al*, 1997). Some clients may be more unpredictable and possibly experience deeper levels of distress, and act out as a means of getting away from having intolerable thoughts or feelings. Indeed, there are some personality disorders, like borderline or histrionic personality disorders, where self-harming is a facet of their personality style. Risk of suicide attempts can be viewed in Box 2.2, which illustrates three main vulnerability factors.

Box 2.2   Vulnerability factors in the risk of suicide

- Poor social support, especially the lack of a confidante
- Inability to respond appropriately to stress
- The presence of a life event (Casey, 1993)

Self-harm needs to be considered in a much wider context than the usual considerations of cutting, burning, head banging or hair pulling. There may be a mixture of self-harming and suicidal tendencies using drugs, alcohol, and/or erratic driving; playing Russian roulette with their lives, leaving it to fate or chance as to whether they will be discovered and saved or undiscovered and die. Self-harm in the form of risk of attack from others may also occur as the client walks alone late at night, works in the sex industry, lives in abusive relationships or gets drunk and picks fights. There is an addictive side to self-harm as the body releases opiates to control pain, which produces feelings of relief or even euphoria; thus it is not easy to stop. In counselling it may be valuable to explore the detail of the self-harming episodes as described in Box 2.3.

Box 2.3   Exploring self-harm episodes

- What is their understanding of what their harming is doing?
- How do they conceal it, or do they do it in front of others?
- What allows them to stop cutting, blood letting or burning?
- Are there abstemious times from self-harming, and what replaces it?
- What does treatment mean to them?
- What helps?

However, sensitivity needs to be exercised, as repetitive self-harmers may find verbal communication difficult, hence the expression through their bodies (Crowe and Bunclark, 2000).

Another risk factor that needs to be considered is medication. The client may be on antipsychotic or antidepressant medication, or a cocktail of such. Some prescribed drugs are dangerous if taken in overdose, like tricyclics or antipsychotics. Selective serotonin reuptake inhibitor (SSRI) antidepressants are not any less of a risk factor for overdosing, because 10 days to 3 weeks after commencing such medication, a very depressed patient may feel sufficiently energised to then attempt suicide. It is therefore sensible to check what is being taken, and discuss medication with the GP, especially if the client is taking antipsychotics and is also using alcohol or recreational drugs, because of interaction effects. Studies suggest that substance misuse occurs in 30–50% of this patient population (George, 2004).

If the client is at risk of self-harm, the counsellor will need to discuss this with the supervisor and/or line manager and the GP. All decision-making processes need to be recorded accurately with the client's counselling notes. Out-of-hours telephone numbers can be provided for the client to place by the phone, e.g. Samaritans or the CMHT emergency numbers. 'Holding' the client, meta-phorically, with keep-safe agreements and delaying tactics until the next session can also provide the impetus for the client to get through the distress and pain of the moment.

Therapeutic models

The Department of Health does not recommend counselling for complex mental health problems or personality disorders (Department of Health, 2001; NICE, 2002). Their approach to therapy with psychosis is to ignore or challenge the voices and what they have to say. However this particular approach may serve to make the client's voices and delusions more entrenched, and may reduce the client's self-esteem.

Person-centred and humanistic methods are non-directive. Therapeutic work may involve engaging the individual in discussion, not with the voices directly, but with the client themselves, perhaps in discussing the process of the voices, the emotional content and the reflection of feelings. Any impact and influence they have on the client as a person may be explored as well as any effect they have on the therapeutic relationship and conversation. Whether the voices are actively trying to inhibit the therapy (Romme and Escher, 1994) may also be addressed. It is empowering to the individual as his or her world of feeling and emotion is acknowledged, helping to relieve any distress. Working with any positive thoughts and 'detoxifying' any negativity associated with the voices can support the client towards a greater sense of self-agency. The aim would be not to remove the voices, but rather to attenuate any associated distress or work with any positive influence that may accompany the voices.

Psychodynamic ways of working with SEMI would focus on the early years of the individual, often building on the object–relation theories of Winnicott (1960) and Klein (1957), the latter arguing that psychotic states are introjective identification and the splitting off from the self. Segel (1957) suggested that the concrete thinking found in psychosis occurs as the individual starts to identify the difference between the self and the object and tries to bridge the two. Rosenfeld (1971, 1987), on the other hand, felt that the psychotic and borderline states could be helped by helping the person to recognise the dependent part of the self that emerges as the childlike state and is often attacked by other aspects of the self.

He argued that the therapist needs to focus on the frustrations and hopelessness within the work that mirror the client's developmental dislocations. Helping the client understand these processes via transference and counter-transference could help the person improve.

Cognitive-behavioural therapy (CBT) for psychosis is a clinically proven method for helping individuals with the distressing positive symptoms of psychosis (Fowler *et al*, 1995; Kingdon and Turkington, 2005). It focuses on the distressing symptoms of the psychosis as well as on the secondary emotional problem. Without patronising patients, it allows them to learn about their difficulties, how and why they arise, and therefore how to alleviate them. It does not aim to change delusional beliefs, or to remove hallucinations, but to reduce the distress caused by preoccupied and obsessive rumination around them. It is known that people's hallucinations tend to be worse when they are anxious or stressed, so looking at their explanations for what is happening to them will affect how distressed they will become. Thus by learning to reframe their experiences with the counsellor's support, they may adopt new strategies for coping.

In a study in North Wales, Startup *et al* (2005) found in a randomly controlled trial that CBT helped people with schizophrenia by reducing positive symptoms which are the acute syndrome, like hallucinations and delusions. Their patients also had fewer negative symptoms, which are the chronic symptoms, like apathy and blunting of affect, and had better social functioning. These benefits had persisted over a two-year period. They also found on a financial cost–benefit analysis that the expense of providing CBT was more than offset by the reduction in cost from people spending less time in hospital.

Working with different disorders

Psychosis is the term used to describe a mental state in which the individual experiences a distortion or loss of contact with reality, in comparison to the neurotic conditions usually presented in primary care, where the individual knows that they feel anxious or depressed and seek help for it.

Schizophrenia

Schizophrenia, schizotypal or psychotic disorders are often described as having three phases: prodromal, active and recovery phases. During the prodromal phase, the client may experience high levels of anxiety, irritability or depression (or rapid shifts between all three). Cognition may be disrupted; there may be deficits in concentration or memory. Thought contents may change as the person becomes preoccupied and ruminates on new ideas. There may be physical changes in sleep, or a loss of energy, and there may be social withdrawal and an inability to do the things the person may normally do. All of these issues are ones that the counsellor may be used to dealing with on a day-to-day level. However, Bentall (2003) suggested that the client's changes in the beliefs about themselves, along with their perceptions and attributions about other people, can change their mood and may precipitate the cascade into a psychosis. The art of good counselling, therefore, is the recognition of such states or 'pre-states', which then becomes prophylactic by preventing the client slipping into the next phase: an active psychotic incident.

The active phase is characterised by the presence of (usually) verbal, auditory hallucinations (like hearing voices), but possibly visual, olfactory or tactile hallucinations as well. There may be unusual or bizarre delusions and/or thoughts manifested by, for example, disintegration of the individual's speech such as 'word salad' (verbigeration). Sometimes psychotic episodes are an expression or re-enactment of past abuse or trauma, so spending time working with the symbolism rather than dismissing them as delusory can allow the client to be heard and valued. So, when working with clients who share information about hearing voices, rather than pathologising the process it may be more meaningful to try and engage with them to discover the symbolic or metaphorical meanings that they contain. Many psychotic symptoms reveal content and, if care is taken to collect a personal history and elicit and listen to the client's 'own personal story', then the counsellor may be in a better position to help the client to identify any patterns and/or repetitions as well as assign any associated personal meaning. For example, the voices or hallucinations that tyrannise the client may be a continuation of what had happened in reality, e.g. the tyranny of an abuser, and thus contribute to a form of post-traumatic stress disorder. In addition, simply listening to a person's 'delusional' experiences, taking them seriously, and allying with the part of the client that has the potential for self-reflection may be helpful, as it can break the isolation often inflicted by psychosis. However, if clients report hearing voices telling them to harm themselves or others, they should be taken seriously. This information should be shared within the primary care team, and a new risk assessment undertaken.

The recovery phase can leave the client feeling vulnerable in the aftermath of the illness. They may be feeling particularly scared, insecure, and uncertain of their future, fearing if or when it will happen again. There may also be grief as they try to resolve the loss of their mental health, the impact on their work and relationships, and the concept of long-term illness and long-term medication.

As previously mentioned, substance misuse is substantially higher in the SEMI population than in the general population (Khalsa *et al*, 1991), and concurrent severe mental health problems and problematic substance misuse is now termed 'dual diagnosis' (Department of Health, 2002). It is also known that for people with predisposition to mental health problems or addiction, the overuse of recreational drugs can precipitate dopamine overactivity, which in turn precipitates psychotic states. Thus, helping with the withdrawal from excessive alcohol or drug use, and breaking down the addictive cycle will be a valuable piece of counselling work. There are also high rates of co-morbid issues, like excessive smoking or obesity, that lead to ongoing physical as well as mental health problems. Mortality rates from cardiovascular and respiratory problems are doubled for patients with schizophrenia (Kendrick, 2004). So helping with lifestyle balance is another valuable piece of work.

For relapse prevention, counsellors should watch for high expressed emotion within families (Leff and Vaughn, 1980). Highly critical and intrusive parents or partners are most likely to provoke a relapse with the client. Therefore, helping the client feel less enmeshed within the family network and developing a secure base for their insecure attachments will minimise the potential for relapse. When working with these clients, it is also important to recognise cultural differences.

We know that men of African–Caribbean origin are three times more likely to receive a diagnosis of schizophrenia than Caucasian men (Littlewood and Lipsedge, 1989). They are more likely to be sectioned under the Mental Health Act, and are more likely to be given higher doses of antipsychotic medication. Yet the cause may be the cultural use of recreational drugs that may make them behave in different ways. In addition, in some cultures, seeing visions or hearing voices is considered a spiritual gift rather than a sign of madness. Cultural religious beliefs in being possessed by demons, the devil, ghosts etc may be wrongly interpreted as delusional beliefs.

Finally, counselling clients with SEMI should not be drastically different from counselling anyone else. They may have multiple problems or needs, but most will be able to prioritise for themselves what they would like to work with in the counselling room. Also, as Bentall (2003) pointed out, the best piece of work may be in working on the acceptance of their mental health differences, as the fear of madness may be greater than the reality of how it is.

Bipolar disorder

Bipolar disorder, or manic depression, affects about 1% of adults during their lifetime. Not all bipolar states are alike, and without intention here to label and with caution against putting individuals into any boxes, it may nevertheless be helpful for those with little or no knowledge of bipolar disorder, to look at the three major forms identified: bipolar I, bipolar II and cyclothymia – although the subcategories may not be the ones routinely used in psychiatric practice.

Cyclothymia is when moods swing from moderately depressed states to mildly manic and back again, and is most likely to be undiagnosed within primary care. Such clients are considered by family members to be moody, unpredictable or petulant. *Bipolar II* clients have much deeper depressive episodes where they feel hopelessness, lose interest in work and life, have reduced libido, and sometimes experience suicidal ideation or attempts, although the manic phase stays moderate. However *bipolar I* clients have the full swing from the most deeply depressed, and very often suicidal, to the highest of mania when people rarely sleep, can become aggressive and impulsive, grandiose, delusory, drive too fast, indulge in indiscriminate sex, spend money wildly or make irrational financial or business decisions. Research has shown that episodes of bipolar swings are unpredictable, and may produce bipolar swings occurring days, weeks or months apart, with no particular sequence of episodes, although it has been noted that the average time between episodes decreases as the number of episodes increases (Post *et al*, 1986).

There tend to be elements of narcissism in an individual who is bipolar, which links in with the grandiosity at times of mania. Schore (1994) suggests that people with bipolar disorder can be disproportionately irritable after mild frustration, readily provoked by seemingly harmless remarks and may react with rage to minor provocations. Some of these individuals may also have developed an ambivalent attachment style, swinging between a needy, preoccupied style, often seen in mania, to an avoidant withdrawal associated with the depression.

More contemporary thinking about bipolar disorder, however, has elucidated the complexity of the bipolar presentation, now called the bipolar spectrum.

This is because bipolar presentation may not necessarily be on a neat continuum between the unipolar depressive state to the bipolar swings of highs or lows. It is now identified that there might be a mixed state of bipolar disorder, where people can experience manic symptoms and depressive symptoms at the same time. This mania can be positive in elation or negative in self-criticism and self-destruction. Or there can be hypomania, where the individual experiences a manic episode without experiencing delusions. The concept of a mood spectrum (Akiskal, 1983) provides a better model for the variety of bipolar presentations, which often may go undiagnosed in primary care.

This concept of bipolar spectrum has been further elaborated into an understanding of 'soft' bipolar disorders (Akiskal, 2003), which are versions of depression without any hypomania, that commonly respond to mood stabilisers but do not respond to antidepressants. These might be people experiencing depressive episodes with co-morbid extreme anxiety, severe insomnia, or extreme irritation with angry outbursts. Morgan (2005) reported on a proposal by Bentall (2003) that mania and depression may not be the opposite ends of an emotional continuum, but that mania may be a psychic defence from the person's desperate attempt to escape from the depressive mood, and what actually fluctuates is the person's self-esteem and positive or negative evaluation of self. Thus the counsellor working on the client's perception of self and self-worth may be valuable in helping the person moderate the swings.

Individuals who have a family member with a mood disorder are at greater risk of developing similar behavioural styles (Kochman et al, 2005). The children of mothers with bipolar disorder may possibly demonstrate a difficulty in regulating their emotions, which can be identified in the child at 12 months old (Gaensbauer et al, 1984), and problems with aggression at 2 years old (Zahn-Waxler et al, 1984). Schore (1994) suggests that this predisposes the child to stress-triggered bipolar illness later in life. This may account for why not all children of manic depressives will also become manic depressives like their parents; there may need to exist an interaction between genetic predisposition and a dysfunctional environment.

Although the more severe forms of the disorder may involve the client being medicated with a mood stabiliser, like lithium, Depakote or carbamazepine, many clients feel unhappy with being held in an artificial stability which gives none of the normal highs and lows of human experience. Indeed, as many people with bipolar disorder are able to access creative aspects of themselves that others cannot attain, some clients are very unwilling to have their creativity taken away by the medication.

Lara et al (2006) have proposed a model that suggests that what underpin the diversity of the presenting mood states are dysregulated fear and anger systems. They argue that fear and anger are an individual's most basic emotions, which initiate or inhibit a person's behaviour. In particular, for many bipolar conditions, the person would have an anger system that is too high, and a fear system that is too low. From a more psychodynamic approach, this model may provide a useful focus for the counselling work, if one concentrates on any dysregulated or accentuated fear or anger states. Counselling with these clients will also involve support through the depressive and self-harming phases, and establishing support networks and keep-safe agreements. It is unlikely that a client will attend for counselling when manic, as the client's grandiosity may pervade and there may be a perception that it is unnecessary as things are 'great'. Afterwards, however, there will be a need for support through the debris of the aftermath of the hurricane of inappropriate and indiscriminate behaviour and risky decision making. In between episodes, some really useful counselling work can be done by focusing on preparation strategies for dealing with the highs and lows: seeking help, developing support networks, and recognising prodromal experiences or triggers and relapse-prevention strategies. Sorensen (2005) has developed a really useful workbook for clients to develop their own relapse-prevention strategies, which can complement the counselling.

Personality disorders

Moran *et al* (1999) conducted research with 303 consecutive primary care patients and found a prevalence rate of personality disorder (PD) of up to 29%. However, as Casey (2000) pointed out, this incidence is likely to be magnified, as people with personality disorder are more frequent attenders of their GP. These patients were also more likely to have a history of psychiatric morbidity, to be single, and to attend the surgery on an emergency basis. As such they can be a considerable burden to the primary care workload.

The signs of a personality disorder usually appear in late childhood or early adolescence and continue into adulthood (in childhood, difficulties experienced are often described as conduct disorders). These individuals have attitudes and behaviours that cause problems for themselves and others. They have a narrow range of (often) dysfunctional coping mechanisms that become entrenched. It is not appropriate to cover the different types of personality disorder in this chapter, and indeed, many individuals fit the criteria for at least two different disorder categories. Most of these individuals are not dangerous, and most will have multiple vulnerabilities and needs. PD may also be a risk indicator for self-harm, as certain types may be characterised by unstable relationships, impulsive and sometimes dangerous behaviour, accompanied by misery and anxiousness. These people are more at risk from suicide attempts, self-harming behaviours and substance abuse.

In the US, the psychoanalytic concept of borderline personality disorder (BPD) provides a rationale for treating these people psychotherapeutically. In the UK, however, psychiatrists are often loath to add them to their workload as there is little proven therapeutic evidence of successful psychiatric treatment. So, large numbers may thus be labelled as 'depressed' and treated with antidepressants (Kendell, 2002). Yet there has recently been very good evidence of successful treatment for personality disorders using cognitive-behavioural methods.

A strategy that can be useful when working with people with personality disorders is to be aware that their difficulties are often synonymous with attachment dysfunction. Commonly, this is a type D attachment style, or disorganised (Lyons-Ruth and Jacobvitz, 1999). These individuals may fail to make or sustain attachments, which in turn may lead to identity confusion as a primary symptom. In addition, they will have little or no sense of boundaries. To escape from the terrifying emptiness and loneliness, they seek closeness with others but then become anxious, as they fear being overwhelmed or invaded by the other. They avoid or fear intimacy, due to fear of repeating past abandonment or rejection episodes, yet paradoxically, they behave to others in ways that are likely to promote abandonment or rejection. Thus working with insecure attachments, which helps the client to learn appropriate emotional distances without acting out the emotional rollercoaster of potential rejection or abandonment, can be enormously beneficial.

The counselling frame, when working with people with a personality disorder, may benefit from being well structured with very strong boundaries, as the client may constantly test these. The counsellor will need to balance empathic recognition of the fear of abandonment with clear boundary setting. For the best effect, the counselling relationship requires a clear focus, and will be relatively long-term, with a strong attachment alliance between the counsellor and client. Clients require frequent risk assessments as they have multiple needs, which can change rapidly. The best support comes from the multiple expertise of a well-integrated primary healthcare team, readily available to the client and the counsellor. Working within the support of a multidisciplinary team can dilute the intensity of the therapeutic work. It can also protect one individual (i.e. the counsellor) from becoming over-involved with a demanding client.

Within the counselling room, clients with personality disorders can often have strong transference reactions (unfortunately, negative therapeutic reactions are frequently common). Indeed, because of their attachment difficulties, there may be difficulty in forming a genuine or deep therapeutic alliance. They may already be well practised at projection, however, so some transference may occur from the outset. If projection onto the therapist is positive, this creates the illusion of a therapeutic alliance, which usually disappears as soon as the counsellor disappoints them, for example, by being unavailable for an appointment (rejection) or going on holiday (abandonment). The counsellor needs to be prepared for equally strong counter-transference reactions (Book, 1997), especially if the counsellor is unprepared for dealing with clients with a borderline or narcissistic personality disorder, where the counsellor will either be the very best or the very worst counsellor in the world. Thus the relationship with the counsellor will become a central issue for the client, and this relationship will be one of the most important relationships in his or her life.

The counsellor's counter-transference reactions, however, need not inhibit therapy, indeed this may be used creatively and carefully, to potentially understand the client in more depth. Thinking about personal responses and analysing them for the information they may be giving about the process of the client can be a helpful experience. For example, if the counsellor feels tempted to help clients by getting them a job, a date, or a home, or the counsellor feels sucked dry, feels the need to withdraw because of her dependence, or feels an overwhelming sense of responsibility, the clients may be showing borderline tendencies. Similarly, if a counsellor feels envy at clients' successes, wonders if she is competent enough to treat them, or feels that she is walking on eggshells because the client may explode with contemptuous rage at minor challenges, the client may be showing narcissistic tendencies. Self-reflection of these issues along with a supervisory discussion may provide insights into the work that was not previously obvious.

Therapeutic ending in general, but especially if premature, with clients with personality disorder can be tricky, as it may tap into abandonment and rejection issues, and a fundamental belief that they are bad and unlovable. So the counsellor would benefit from being very clear with clients that an ending of a short-term contract is not their fault, and they did not fail in therapy. Splitting can be discouraged by engaging the client in a discussion about the therapy experience as a whole, as suggested in Box 2.4, and then moving on to discuss what might happen next.

Box 2.4   Discouraging 'splitting' when ending with a client with personality disorder

- What did he/she like/not like about it?
- What did he/she like/not like about you?
- What did he/she achieve?
- What was disappointing?

Preferably, a referral will be made to an alternative therapist, if appropriate, before these discussions take place, so that the client does not feel left isolated and alone, enhancing the process of ending.

Conclusion

Counselling with people with SEMI can be a rewarding experience as one facilitates the client's progress from a potentially dysfunctional 'severe' state or 'enduring' way of life, to hopefully a more functional, meaningful state of wellbeing. It may also be challenging as the counsellor tries to unpack the breadth and depth of the client's often very deep personal trauma. Burton and Davey (1996) suggested that this more complex client group, often considered 'heart-sink' patients, unfortunately tends to be allocated to counsellors with little experience with this population in NHS settings. They suggested that this may be because more experienced mental health professionals would prefer not to work with these individuals, as they know how hard it can get. Consequently, working with a multidisciplinary primary healthcare team is the best-case scenario, as the team supports the distribution of the intensity of the therapeutic alliance, and prevents the counsellor from being the client's only 'safe base'. Working with ongoing supportive supervision or peer consultation with someone who is familiar with the processes of SEMI is essential to support the counsellor from becoming over-burdened and to help maintain clear boundaries. Furthermore, as was mentioned previously, since emotional stress is common generally, and counter-transference reactions may be common specifically, ongoing personal therapy and supervision will help counsellors to distinguish between the client's and their own material. Finally, overall, clients with SEMI may provide a challenge for the counsellor, and likewise can equally be extremely rewarding.

References

Akiskal HS (1983) The bipolar spectrum: new concepts in classification and diagnosis. In: Grinspoon L (ed.) *Psychiatry Update: the American Psychiatric Association Annual Review* Vol. 2. Washington DC: American Psychiatric Press, pp. 271–92.

Akiskal HS (2003) Validating 'hard' and 'soft' phenotypes within the bipolar spectrum: continuity or discontinuity? *Journal of Affective Disorder* 73:1–5.

Bak M, Krabbendam L, Janssen I *et al* (2005) Early trauma may increase the risk for psychotic experiences by impacting on emotional response and perception of control. *Acta Psychiatrica Scandinavia* 112:360–6.

Barr W (2000) *Do Severe and Enduring Mental Illness (SEMI) Registers in Primary Health Care (PHC) Make a Difference?* Summary number 568. The Research Findings Register. London: Department of Health.

Bentall R (2003) *Madness Explained*. London: Allen Lane/Penguin.

Book HE (1997) Countertransference and the difficult personality-disordered patient. In: Rosenbluth M (ed.) *Treating Difficult Personality Disorders*. San Francisco: Wiley, pp. 173–203.

Burton M and Davey T (1996) The psychodynamic paradigm. In: Woolfe R and Dryden W (eds) *Handbook of Counselling Psychology*. London: Sage, pp. 113–32.

Casey P (1993) Social function in adult psychiatric disorders. In: Tyrer P and Casey P (eds) *Social Function in Psychiatry: the hidden axis of classification*. Petersfield: Wrightson Biomedical Publishing, pp. 71–84.

Casey P (2000) The epidemiology of personality disorder. In: Tyrer P (ed.) *Personality Disorders. Diagnosis, management and course* (2e). Oxford: Butterworth-Heinemann, pp. 71–9.

Crowe M and Bunclark J (2000) Self injury: a struggle. *International Review of Psychiatry* 12:48–53.

Department of Health (2001) *Treatment Choice in Psychological Therapies and Counselling. Evidence based clinical practice guideline*. London: Department of Health.

Department of Health (2002) *Mental Health Policy. Implementation guide. Dual diagnosis good practice guide*. London: Department of Health.

Fowler D, Garety P and Kuipers E (1995) *Cognitive Behaviour Therapy for Psychosis. Theory and practice*. Chichester: Wiley.

Gaensbauer TJ, Harmon RJ, Cytryn L and McKnew DH (1984) Differences in the patterning of affective expression in infants. *Journal of the American Academy of Child Psychiatry* 141:223–9.

George M (2004) People with mental health problems. *Care and Health*. 17 December 2003–6 January 2004.

Kendell RE (2002) The distinction between personality disorder and mental illness. *British Journal of Psychiatry* 180:110–15.

Kendler KS, Bulik CM, Silberg J *et al* (2000) Childhood sexual abuse and adult psychiatric and substance use disorders in women. An epidemiological and Cotwin control analysis. *Archives of General Psychiatry* 57:953–9.

Kendrick T (2004) The role of the general practitioner in severe mental illness. *Psychiatry* 3:26–8.

Khalsa HK, Shamer A and Anglin MD (1991) The prevalence of substance abuse in a psychiatric evaluation unit. *Drug and Alcohol Dependence* 28:215–23.

Kingdon D and Turkington D (2005) *Cognitive Therapy of Schizophrenia*. New York: Guilford Press.

Klein M (1957) *The Writings of Melanie Klein*. London: Hogarth Press.

Kochman FJ, Hantouche EG, Ferrari P *et al* (2005) Cyclothymic temperament as a prospective predictor of bipolarity and suicidality in children and adolescents with major depressive disorder. *Journal of Affective Disorders* 85:181–9.

Lara DR, Pinto O, Akiskal K and Akiskal HS (2006) Toward an integrative model of the spectrum of mood, behavioural and personality disorders based on fear and anger traits: I. Clinical implications. *Journal of Affective Disorders* 94:67–87.

Leff JP and Vaughn C (1980) The interaction of life-events and relatives' expressed emotion in schizophrenia and depressive neurosis. *British Journal of Psychiatry* 136:146–53.

Littlewood R and Lipsedge M (1989) *Aliens and Alienists: ethnic minorities and psychiatry* (2e). London: Unwin Hyman.

Lyons-Ruth K and Jacobvitz D (1999) Attachment Disorganisation. Unresolved loss, relational violence, and lapses in behavioural attentional strategies. In: Cassidy J and Shaver PR (eds) *Handbook of Attachment. Theory, research, and clinical applications.* New York: The Guilford Press, pp. 520–54.

Mental After Care Association (MACA) (1999) *First National GP Survey of Mental health in Primary Care.* London: Mental After care Association, Partners in Mental Health in England and Scotland.

Maher BA (1988) Delusions as the product of normal cognitions. In: Oltmanns TF and Maher BA (eds) *Delusional Beliefs.* Oxford: Wiley, pp. 333–6.

Moran P, Jenkins R, Mann A and Tylee A (1999) Personality disorder in primary care. *Current Opinion in Psychiatry* 12(Suppl. 1):140.

Morgan J (2005) Ups and downs in bipolar disorder. *The Psychologist* 18:346.

National Institute for Clinical Excellence (2002) *Schizophrenia. Core interventions in the treatment and management of schizophrenia in primary and secondary care.* London: National Institute for Clinical Excellence.

Post RM, Rubinow DR and Ballenger JC (1986) Conditioning and sensitization in the longitudinal course of affective illness. *British Journal of Psychiatry* 149:191–201.

Read J (2005) The bio-bio-bio model of madness. *The Psychologist* 18:596–7.

Read J, Mosher L and Bentall R (2004) *Models of Madness.* Hove: Brunner-Routledge.

Romme M and Escher S (1994) *Accepting Voices.* London: Mind Publications.

Rosenfeld H (1971) A clinical approach to the psychoanalytic theory of the life and death instincts: an investigation into the aggressive aspects of narcissism. *International Journal of Psycho-Analysis* 52:169–78.

Rosenfeld H (1987) *Impasse and Interpretation.* London: Tavistock.

Russello A (2004) SEMI trained . . . or not? *Healthcare Counselling and Psychotherapy Journal* 4(1):2–5.

Schore A (1994) *Affect Regulation and the Development of the Self.* New Jersey: Lawrence Erlbaum.

Segel H (1957) Notes on symbol formation. *International Journal of Psycho-Analysis* 38:391–7.

Slade M, Powell R and Strathdee G (1997) Current approaches to identifying the severely mentally ill. *Social Psychiatry and Psychiatric Epidemiology* 32:177–84.

Sorensen J (2005) *Relapse Prevention in Bipolar Disorder. A treatment manual and workbook for therapist and client.* Hatfield: University of Hertfordshire Press.

Startup M, Jackson MC, Evans KE and Bendix S (2005) North Wales randomised controlled trial of cognitive behaviour therapy for acute schizophrenia spectrum disorders: two-year follow-up and economic evaluation. *Psychological Medicine* 35:1307–16.

Teicher MH (2002) Scars that won't heal: the neurobiology of child abuse. *Scientific American* 286:54–61.

Tien AY (1991) Distribution of hallucinations in the population. *Social and Psychiatric Epidemiology* 26:287–92.

Winnicott DW (1960) The theory of parent–infant relationship. *International Journal of Psycho-Analysis* 41:585–95.

Zahn-Waxler C, McKnew DH, Cummings M, Davenport WB and Radke-Yarrow M (1984) Problem behaviours and peer interaction of young children with a manic-depressive parent. *American Journal of Psychiatry* 141:236–40.

Chapter 3

Understanding mental health and mental illness

April Russello

Introduction

This chapter discusses the concepts of mental health and mental ill-health; it explains the mental state examination (a way of eliciting symptoms and structuring the information elicited or observed, in relation to an individual's mental health) and identifies some of the causes and vulnerability/protective factors that can affect mental health. The terms mental disorder and illness are used interchangeably. It is hoped that this chapter will encourage readers to reflect on their understanding of mental health and illness.

Concepts of mental health and mental illness

The concept of 'mental illness' has little meaning without a concept of mental health against which one may measure or gauge mental illness. Good mental health is not merely an absence of illness or disorder but 'includes a positive sense of wellbeing; individual resources including self-esteem, optimism, a sense of mastery and coherence; the ability to initiate, develop and sustain mutually satisfying personal relationships and the ability to cope with adversities' (Jenkins *et al*, 2001, p. xvi). Moreover, it is probably a common misconception to view mental health and mental illness as dichotomous. Rather, they may best be understood as different points on a continuum; a continuum one hastens to add, on which each and every one of us can be found at different points, at different times in our lives, for different reasons.

Most people experience some small or large difficulties or problems at one time or another during the course of their life. This may cause an individual to endure stress and/or distress and possibly some physical or mental dysfunction. Mentally healthy people may not always be happy, every day and all of the time. Everyone's life will usually, inevitably, contain some discomfort or sorrow; yet also, paradoxically, very happy events, as well as the 'usual' sad life events, can trigger the subsequent appearance of minor physical and/or psychological 'symptoms' and/or dysfunction.

The very concept of 'normal' is of limited usefulness since it frequently varies between cultures, generations and countries. Indeed, it is a commonly held belief that 'we are all a little mad' (Clare, 1976). In a paper on schizoid factors in the personality, Fairbairn, in 1940, made the following statement which still seems perfectly applicable today:

> *according to my way of thinking, everybody without exception must be regarded as schizoid. The fundamental schizoid phenomenon is the presence of splits in the ego; and it would take a bold man to claim that his ego was so perfectly integrated as to be incapable of splitting at the deepest levels, or that such evidence of splitting of the ego could in no circumstances declare itself at more superficial levels, even under conditions of extreme suffering or hardship or deprivation.*

A common language

Mental health and other professionals often use a particular terminology like GP (general practitioner) and CPN (community psychiatric nurse) and LTD (long-term depression). This can be helpful since it enables healthcare professionals to 'speak a common language' as well as offering clients and patients hope for understanding the subjective distress that frequently accompanies a mental health problem. It also enables them to receive appropriate treatment and support. It may unfortunately, however, seem to 'label' and stigmatise. The acronym SEMI for example is a 'shorthand' way of describing severe and enduring mental illness; unhappily, however, it may also convey the idea of something or someone being 'semi' i.e. partially or not quite complete. While such associations are regrettable, when used sensitively and respectfully, then practitioners can communicate in this 'shorthand' form verbally and in writing, and most importantly can spend more time in actual practice with clients and patients.

Box 3.1 offers a selection of commonly used mental health terms that can be useful to know. Mental disorders are classified into diagnostic categories that are defined in terms of patterns of signs and symptoms, the course the disorder takes and its 'usual' outcome. Every disorder has its own characteristic pattern which may vary slightly between individuals. Signs and symptoms of mental disorders usually occur in recognisable patterns that are called syndromes. Bipolar depression for example, which is considered a SEMI, follows a pattern of episodic mood swings between mania or elevated mood and depression or low mood. One may observe *signs* of activity or restlessness and hear about delusional thinking from the client/patient, while the individual themselves may report *symptoms* of insomnia or auditory hallucinations.

Understanding the commonly used terms in mental health can facilitate understanding between different professionals from different disciplines, making communication more effective and efficient. 'It's all about learning the language even if one doesn't like it or agree with the concepts of psychiatry' (Freeth and Knowles, 2006).

Box 3.1   Selected mental health terms

- *Sign*: what the therapist or other clinician has observed or elicited; signs may not be apparent to the client or patient
- *Symptom*: a subjective indicator of a disorder noticed by the client or patient

- *Syndrome*: a collection of signs and symptoms that frequently occur in recognisable patterns forming a distinct clinical picture indicative of a particular disorder
- *Delusion*: a false belief held with absolute conviction which is not affected by logical argument or a conventionally held belief, due to one's cultural or educational background
- *Hallucination*: a false perception in any of the senses in the absence of any external stimuli
- *Mental Disorder*: '. . . a clinically recognisable set of symptoms or behaviours associated in most cases with distress and with interference with personal function. Social deviance or conflict alone, without personal dysfunction should not be included in mental disorder' (World Health Organization, 1992)
- *Discriminating symptoms*: symptoms commonly found in a particular syndrome, but rarely in other syndromes
- *Characteristic symptoms*: symptoms that occur frequently in a particular syndrome but also in others
- *Depersonalisation*: when an individual feels unreal, lifeless
- *Derealisation*: when an individual experiences others as unreal, lifeless

The human mental state

Throughout life, one's mental health will have an effect on one's thinking, feeling, behaviour, cognitions, and perceptions, about oneself and towards others. Recognising mental health problems depends on the healthcare practitioner's skills of observation and listening and the ability to elicit information through questioning about a client's or a patient's mental state. Box 3.2 illustrates the basic contents of the human mental state. These are the domains in which the mind functions and where mental dysfunction occurs and may frequently be observed.

Box 3.2   Basic contents of a mental state

- *Behaviour*: actions and external manifestations of the internal mental state
- *Thoughts*: ideas, concepts, the inner dialogue with oneself
- *Emotions*: subjective feeling–states, e.g. happiness, anger or sadness
- *Cognitions*: the basic abilities of intelligence–attention, concentration, memory, calculation, language
- *Perceptions*: the functioning of the five sensory modalities: touch, hearing, taste, sight and smell

---

One of the ways of eliciting information about possible mental disorder is through a mental state examination (MSE). The MSE provides a useful organisational framework for eliciting signs and symptoms of mental health and mental disorder in a systematic fashion. The MSE is part of the history taken by psychiatrists when a patient is referred to them. Using the MSE, however, does not imply that the mental health practitioner is trying to be a psychiatrist, nor does it entitle one to make a diagnosis; it is basically a handy tool that can help the practitioner structure one's thoughts with regard to mental health. Knowledge of the MSE and awareness of the manifestations of an individual's mental state can enable practitioners to be more informed in relation to what is elicited or being observed. It may be helpful simply to keep the content of the MSE in mind when meeting a client or patient for the first time. Some areas of the MSE, such as appearance and behaviour, rely on observation, whereas other areas, beliefs for example, will need to be elicited.

Box 3.3 illustrates the content of the MSE; the aim is to assess the state of mind *at the time the interview or session is being conducted*. Areas to observe or inquire about are provided in brief, following the categories for examination which are in italics. Of course culture, education and religion of the client or patient must be taken into consideration, since for example some individuals may avoid eye contact because in their culture it would be considered rude or immodest to sustain direct eye contact.

Box 3.3   The mental state examination

- *Appearance and behaviour*: what is the individual's general appearance, is there eye contact, self-care, posture, motor activity, movement . . . is it overly slow or fast?
- *Speech*: how is the person speaking, at what rate, quantity, pattern, is there continuity to their ideas?
- *Thought*: what is the content, are there any preoccupations, obsessions, over-valued ideas, delusions, suicidal thoughts?
- *Mood*: this is subjective, as expressed by the client. What is the prevailing mood, any variations, is it congruent or incongruent with what they are saying (an example of possible incongruence might be saying they are sad while laughing or smiling)?
- *Affect*: this is what is observed. Are there any external manifestations of emotion, e.g. laughter, tears?
- *Abnormal experiences*: do they relate any sense of depersonalisation or derealisation?
- *Beliefs*: are there any delusions?
- *Perception*: are there any hallucinations?
- *Cognition*: what is their sense of orientation (of time, place and person), how are their attention (ability to focus) and concentration (capacity to sustain that focus) and memory (long/short term)?
- *Insight*: do they believe that they are ill, how aware do they seem to be about what they are saying or presenting and to what do they attribute their symptoms?

If one is uncertain about what the client or patient is presenting, knowledge of the *discriminating symptoms* and *characteristic symptoms* of the different mental disorders can help distinguish between the different conditions. For example, thought insertion (a delusion of thoughts being inserted into one's mind) is a discriminating symptom of schizophrenia, while suicidal thoughts would be considered a characteristic symptom because they can occur in several other kinds of mental disorders.

Knowledge of mental health and use of some of the tools such as the MSE, do not mean that one must subscribe to a medical model or any particular theoretical or philosophical orientation. A counsellor or psychotherapist or any healthcare professional may, through knowledge of the MSE, enhance their ability to recognise their clients' and patients' mental health problems without compromising a person-centred way of working. Basic knowledge of mental health, mental illness and familiarity with the mental disorders listed in the psychiatric diagnostic manuals *International Classification of Disease (ICD-10)* (World Health Organization, 1992; see Box 3.4) and the *DSM IV* (American Psychiatric Association, 2000) can make a difference to healthcare practitioners' practice and to clients or patients; indeed 'it is essential to be familiar with psychiatry's diagnostic manuals ICD10 and DSM . . .' (Freeth and Knowles, 2006).

Box 3.4   Main diagnostic categories in *ICD-10*

- Organic disorders including dementia, delirium and amnesiac syndromes
- Mental and behavioural disorders due to psychoactive substance abuse, e.g. due to use of alcohol, volatile substances (for example glue) or hallucinogens
- Schizophrenia (including schizotypal, delusional and other psychotic disorders)
- Mood (affective) disorders (uni-polar, i.e. only depression/low mood; and bipolar, i.e. episodes of both elevation of mood – mania – *and* depression)
- Neurotic, stress-related and somatoform disorders; includes obsessive–compulsive disorder
- Behavioural syndromes associated with physiological disturbances and physical factors, e.g. eating disorders
- Disorders of adult personality and behaviour, e.g. specific personality disorders such as paranoid personality disorder
- Mental retardation: usually divided into mild, moderate and severe
- Disorders of psychological development, e.g. childhood autism
- Behavioural and emotional disorders with onset usually occurring in childhood and adolescence, e.g. conduct disorders
- Unspecified mental disorders

These are the main *ICD-10* categories, please consult the *ICD-10* (World Health Organization, 1992) for further information and the subcategories.

Vulnerability and protective factors impacting on mental health

Life events such as marriage, divorce, death, childbirth and similar important occasions, are times of transition and may precipitate emotional difficulties. Similarly, factors such as loss of a parent in childhood may predispose an individual to become more vulnerable to emotional difficulties or disorders. Furthermore, there may be issues that perpetuate an individual's emotional problem or disorder. These three factors, also known as 'the three Ps' and listed in Box 3.5, can have an influential effect on an individual's mental health. Inquiry into these three areas can help structure and guide the questions the practitioner asks, particularly in the initial meeting, but the 'three Ps' are also useful to bear in mind when exploring most problems or difficulties in general.

Mental health problems are often the result of the complex interaction of biological, social and personal factors. Some individuals may be biologically vulnerable to depression, yet good social support throughout difficult times may decrease their risk of becoming depressed, for example. Similarly, psychotic episodes may be triggered by stressful life events and circumstances, in individuals with a high genetic risk of schizophrenia.

Box 3.5   The 'three Ps' inquiry factors and select examples

Precipitating events

These are events that occur just prior to the onset of a problem, difficulty or disorder such as: *hyperventilation; side-effects of medication; stressful or significant life events; muscular tension; physical pathology*

Predisposing factors

These may be: *genetics; early life events; early family dynamics; socio-economic factors; the individual's overall personality; beliefs about illness and illness causation*

Perpetuating factors

These are factors that prolong the course of a difficulty or problem and can undermine the return of mental health and wellbeing, for example: *lack of a confidante; ongoing physical illness; environmental factors; dysfunctional family relationships*

Further factors associated with having an impact on mental health include the following:

Environment

The environment in which our clients or patients live or work may have an effect on their mental health. Poor living conditions are commonly supposed to predispose to mental ill-health (Freeman, 1984) whether as a direct impact or because of their effects on relationships or family life. Noise (Jenkins *et al*, 1981) is another environmental factor that is suggested to have an impact on mental health, although the evidence is inconclusive. Unsurprisingly perhaps, prolonged unemployment (Banks and Jackson, 1982; Warr and Jackson, 1985) has also been considered a factor affecting mental health; there may be confounding variables, however, because unemployment may lead to a poor living environment. Similarly, one could argue that social inequalities could lead to substance abuse, which in some cases could be responsible for the development of anxiety or depressive disorders. In addition, working conditions may also impact on mental health (Broadbent, 1981).

Life events

Although an association between life events and illness does not automatically indicate causality, periods of life changes (Rahe *et al*, 1970) for both good and bad are associated with illness. 'Exit events' or events involving loss or departure of an individual from the immediate social field of the client or patient, are loosely associated with depression (Paykel *et al*, 1969). Creed (1992), writing about 'life events', looked at two studies on life events in depression and schizophrenia using the 'Life-Events and Difficulties Schedule' (LEDS). In the study on schizophrenia, following a relapse, there was a clear increase in subjects experiencing life events prior to relapse when compared with a control group, *even if the life events were relatively minor and non-threatening*. In the study on depression conducted with women participants, only events with a severe threat were common among the depressed group and not mild or non-threatening events. This seems to suggest that individuals with schizophrenia may perceive life events, however minor or non-threatening, as disruptive, severe and threatening.

Vulnerability and protective factors

This means that individual attributes to any given life event will inevitably vary between people according to their past experiences, so people experiencing the same event will most likely have quite different responses. Certain factors, however, may increase vulnerability to life events, whereas other factors may offer protection against such events. An example of a vulnerability factor is having the care of several small children; whereas a protective factor is having a confidante, such as a spouse or partner (Brown and Harris, 1978).

In their Camberwell study conducted with inner-city women, Brown and Harris (1978) identified the four vulnerability factors shown in Box 3.6 associated with this group.

Box 3.6   Four vulnerability factors (Brown and Harris, 1978)

- Lack of a confiding relationship
- Three or more children under the age of 14, living at home
- Not having employment outside of the home
- Loss of mother around the age of eleven years old

Conclusion

The concepts of mental health and mental disorder are not clear-cut, they do not stand on opposite ends of a pole, like 'yes–no'; 'up–down'; 'right–wrong'; 'black–white'; the concept of 'normal' is indeed a very 'grey' area needing careful, sensitive, consideration and assessment when attempting to ascertain a mental state. Mental health is an important factor when seeking to understand mental ill-health because it does not mean merely an absence of symptoms; over time, low self-esteem and low self-confidence, general pessimism and lack of any relationships, may erode an individual's mental health.

In the 'world of mental health' and psychiatry, many different and specific words and terms are used which may in fact be quite disagreeable to many practitioners. This may also include psychiatrists such as Rachel Freeth who, in Chapter 7 of this book, expresses concerns about the language of acronyms and jargon that can seem to reduce individuals to terms and numbers instead of human beings. There are many abbreviations and terms that seem confusing and puzzling or can seem downright negative. This emphasises the need to use these carefully and with sensitivity, without which, the language may dehumanise both patients and practitioners.

Many practitioners find themselves in the situation of trying to gauge their client's or patient's mental health, and it may sometimes need to be done sooner rather than later. Knowledge of the content of the MSE, in such specific times as well as in general, can be an extremely useful tool to bear in mind. Of course this does not enable non-medical practitioners to make diagnoses; it can, however, help ensure that the practitioner accesses information in a systematic way, making them more informed and thus better able to provide effective help or appropriate referral.

Similarly, knowledge of the 'three Ps' and the factors that are associated with mental health and illness can assist the practitioner in their aim to help their clients and patients.

Finally, although it may seem obvious, individuals are just that, individuals; each of us is different and we respond differently to life and what it brings us. There is no 'one size fits all' in mental health. This chapter is meant to invite readers to think about and reflect on their own understanding and recognition of individuals' mental health and illness, as well as the way we practise. This chapter embodies and reveals this writer's approach, and ideas and concepts that have been helpful and influential in my own practice; perhaps they might also be, in yours?

Acknowledgements

Many thanks to Maggie Pettifer for her support and for encouraging the writing of this book. A very big thank you to the director of my PhD studies, Professor Joan Curzio, whose patience and trust have been a beacon, and finally my grateful thanks to my co-authors who put up with my endless requests and ceaseless 'gentle reminders', and who never, ever, let me down.

Further reading

Gamble C and Brennan G (2000) *Working with Serious Mental Illness; A Manual for Clinical Practice*. London: Balliere Tindall.

Jongsma AE and Berghuis DJ (2000) *The Severe and Persistent Mental Illness Treatment Planner*. New York: J Wiley & Sons.

Jenkins R, McCulloch A, Friedli L and Parker C (2001) *Maudsley Monographs 434. Developing a National Mental Health Policy*. Hove: Psychology Press Ltd.

World Health Organization (2004) *WHO Guide to Mental and Neurological Health in Primary Care* (2e). Geneva: World Health Organization.

References

American Psychiatric Association (2000) *DSM IV American Psychiatric Association Diagnostic and Statistical Manual of Mental Disorders* (4e). Washington DC: American Psychiatric Association.

Banks MH and Jackson PR (1982) Unemployment and Risk of Minor Psychiatric Disorder in Young People: cross sectional and longitudinal evidence. *Psychological Medicine* 12:789–98.

Broadbent DE (1981) Chronic Affects From the Physical Nature of Work. In: Gardell B and Johnson G (eds) *Working Life: a social science contribution to work reform*. Chichester: Wiley, pp. 39–51.

Brown GW and Harris TO (1978) *Social Origins of Depression*. London: Tavistock Publications Ltd.

Clare A (1976) *Psychiatry in Dissent; Controversial Issues in Thought and Practice*. London: Tavistock Publications Ltd.

Creed F (1992) Life events. In: Weller M and Eysenck M (eds) *The Scientific Basis of Psychiatry* (2e). London: Saunders Company Limited, pp. 491–508.

Fairbairn WRD (1940) *Schizoid Factors in the Personality; Psychoanalytic Studies of the Personality*. London: Routledge and Kegan Paul, pp. 3–27. (An abbreviated version of this paper was read before the Scottish branch of the British Psychological Society on 9 November 1940.)

Freeman H (ed.) (1984) *Mental Health and the Environment*. Edinburgh: Churchill Livingstone.

Freeth R and Knowles (2006) In interview by Pointon C: Gulfs and Bridges; is it possible to cut the stereotypical ribbon and open a highway between the worlds of counselling/psychotherapy and psychiatry? *Therapy Today* 17(4).

Jenkins L, Tarnopolsky A and Hand D (1981) Psychiatric admissions and aircraft noise from London Airport: four year, three hospitals' study. *Psychological Medicine* 11(4):765–82.

Jenkins R, McCulloch A, Friedli L and Parker C (2001) *Maudsley Monographs 434. Developing a National Mental Health Policy*. Hove: Psychology Press Ltd.

Paykel ES, Myers JK, Deinelt MN *et al* (1969) Life events and depression; a controlled study. *Archives of General Psychiatry* 21:753–60.

Rahe R, Gunderson EKE and Arthur RJ (1970) Demographic and psychosocial factors in acute illness reporting. *Journal of Chronic Diseases* 23:245–55.

Warr P and Jackson P (1985) Factors influencing the psychological impact of prolonged unemployment and re-employment. *Psychological Medicine* 15:795–808.

World Health Organization (1992). *ICD-10 Classification of Mental and Behavioural Disorders Clinical Descriptions and Diagnostic Guidelines*. Geneva: World Health Organization.

Individuals with severe and enduring mental illness, and the role of primary care

Helen Lester

Introduction

This chapter explores the potential roles and responsibilities of the primary care team in the care of people with serious and enduring mental illness. The scope is deliberately broad, emphasising the very different needs of the young person walking through the door with difficult-to-detect symptoms of first-episode psychosis (FEP) and the adult with a diagnosis of psychosis who has been unemployed for decades. The value and meaning of shared care will be discussed, and users' views, key to understanding the role of primary care, will also be explored. The influence of mental health policy on the way we practise will be an underpinning theme throughout the chapter.

How involved is primary care with people with severe and enduring mental illness?

Serious mental illness can be difficult to define. If people with schizophrenia, bipolar disorder and chronic psychosis are included, it affects 3% of the population in the UK (Bird, 1999). In the UK, people with SEMI consult primary care practitioners more frequently (Nazareth *et al*, 1993) and are in contact with primary care services for a longer cumulative time than patients without mental health problems (Lang *et al*, 1997; Kai *et al*, 2000). Indeed, 30–50% of people with SEMI are seen only in the primary care setting (Jenkins *et al*, 2002), that is, the 'front line' of the health service staffed predominantly by GPs and practice nurses supported by a legion of others professionals including counsellors, chiropodists and physiotherapists. However, despite the prevalence and, in the UK at least, the considerable use people with SEMI make of primary care services, many GPs still feel that, in contrast to patients with complex diabetes or heart failure for example, holistic care of patients with SEMI is beyond their remit. The majority regard themselves as involved in the monitoring and treatment of mental illness (Kendrick *et al*, 1991; Bindman *et al*, 1997; Burns *et al*, 2000). There is also some evidence that people with SEMI are perceived as 'difficult' and as creating work, with the attitudes of inner-city GPs being particularly negative (Brown *et al*,

1999a). Two UK studies compared patients with and without a diagnosis of schizophrenia and found that the patients with schizophrenia were more likely to encounter reluctance by GPs to participate in their care and be referred to a hospital specialist (Lawrie *et al*, 1996, 1998). This, of course, may well reflect the negative stereotypes held by many in wider society, or at the very least, a perception of 'otherness', evocatively described by Jonathan Miller:

> *There is a vast and very complicated unwritten constitution of conduct which allows us to move with confidence through public spaces, and we can instantly and by a very subtle process recognise someone who is breaking that constitution. They are talking to themselves; they are not moving at the same rate; they are moving at different angles; they are not avoiding other people with the skills that pedestrians do in the street. The speed, with which normal users of public places can recognise someone else as not being a normal user of it, is where madness appears.*

(Miller, 1991, pp. 6–7.)

GPs' relative lack of enthusiasm and involvement may also reflect a paucity of formal training in mental health in the UK. A recent survey found that only one-third of GPs had received any mental health training in the last five years, while 10% expressed concerns about their training or skills needs in mental health (Mental After Care Association, 1999). Mental health issues are, of course, also a significant part of the workload of many practice nurses. A national survey of practice nurse involvement in mental health interventions found that 51% were administering depots (injections of antipsychotic drugs) at least once a month, 33% were involved in ensuring compliance with antipsychotic medication, and 30% with monitoring side-effects of medication (Gray *et al*, 1999). Despite this, few practice nurses have had specific training in mental health issues. Only 2% of practice nurses have had dedicated mental health training and, in a survey published in 1999, up to 70% of practice nurses reported receiving no mental health training at all in the previous five years (Gray *et al*, 1999). It is therefore perhaps unsurprising that many practice nurses report a lack of confidence in their ability to talk to and treat people with mental health problems (Crosland and Kai, 1998). However, practice nurses do have considerable transferable experience, for example in running specialist clinics for patients with chronic physical health problems that incorporate systematic assessment of symptoms, treatment effects and side-effects, the use of protocols for modifying management, and proactive follow-up of non-attendees. These are skills that have made them key in achieving new GP contract targets (*see* later in this chapter, p. 41).

Patients with SEMI, however, require, if anything, a better standard of primary care than the general population (Connolly and Kelly, 2005). A meta-analysis by Harris and Barraclough (1998) looked at mortality rates in people with severe mental illness. They analysed 20 papers, covering a population of 36 000 people from nine countries, that related specifically to schizophrenia. Using these data they calculated standardised mortality rates (SMRs) for this group as a whole, and for specific causes of death. The SMR for males with schizophrenia for all causes of death was 156 (95% confidence interval (CI) 151–162) and for females with schizophrenia it was 141 (95% CI 136–146). The SMR for infectious diseases as a cause of death in people with schizophrenia was 455 for males and 490 for females. The SMR for respiratory diseases causing death was 214 for males and

249 for females. More recently, the Office of National Statistics survey *Psychiatric Morbidity among Adults Living in Private Households* (Singleton *et al*, 2001) found that 62% of people with psychosis reported a physical condition, compared to 42% of those without a psychosis. Diabetes, for example, is up to five times as frequent in patients with schizophrenia or bipolar affective disorder, as in the general population (Mukherjee *et al*, 1996).

There are a number of possible reasons for these statistics, including lifestyle, diet, physical activity, smoking, obesity, drug side-effects and a relative lack of healthcare promotion and prevention. Brown *et al* (1999b) prospectively surveyed the lifestyles of 140 people with schizophrenia, and found that their diet was unhealthy (higher in fat and lower in fibre than the reference population), they took less exercise than the reference population, and also had significantly higher levels of cigarette smoking (90% of people with schizophrenia and about 30% of people with bipolar disorder smoke) (Brown *et al*, 1999b). A number of psychotropic drugs have a high risk of cardiotoxicity, with potentially harmful effects on electrophysiology and myocardial function (Chong *et al*, 2001). Haematological complications can also occur (Oyesanmi *et al*, 1999). Phenothiazines, and the newer atypical antipsychotics have also been shown to increase both central obesity, and to be associated with diabetes (Sernyak *et al*, 2002).

There is also evidence that health-promotion activities in primary care are different for people with and without SEMI. Burns and Cohen (1998) found that although the annual general practice consultation rate was significantly higher than normal for people with SEMI (13–14 consultations a year compared to approximately three for the general population), the amount of data recorded for a range of health-promotion areas was significantly less than in consultations with people without SEMI. Cardiovascular risk factors in particular were less likely to be recorded in primary care records or acted upon than in the general population (Kendrick, 1996). A recent interim report by the Disability Rights Commission based on the primary care records of 1.7 million primary care patients also found that women with schizophrenia were less likely to have had a cervical smear in the previous five years (63%) compared to the general population (73%), and that 68% of people with schizophrenia and heart disease had had a recent cholesterol test compared with 80% of the remaining population with heart disease (Disability Rights Commission, 2005). We are therefore left with a situation where people with SEMI require particularly good primary care, yet appear, for a variety of reasons, to not always receive it.

Primary care and the initial diagnosis of psychosis

Early intervention in psychosis is a relatively new concept in mental health. It describes the health service and wider policy response to the increasing evidence of an unacceptably long duration of untreated psychosis (DUP), i.e. the time interval between the onset of psychotic symptoms and the start of antipsychotic treatment, and the benefits of early diagnosis and treatment for young people experiencing an FEP. Eighty per cent of FEPs occur in young people between 16 and 30 years of age, at a critical time in their intellectual and social development and emerging personal autonomy. Studies across the world on FEP have consistently found an average DUP of one to two years (McGlashan, 1999). Such delays would be unacceptable in physical illness, where a maximum two-week wait for suspected cancer referrals and two-hour 'pain to needle' thrombolysis targets in suspected myocardial infarctions are part of standard care in the UK.

Although still somewhat disputed, it is highly likely that an association exists between DUP and outcome in FEP, particularly functional and symptomatic outcome at 12 months and symptom reduction once treatment begins (Harrigan *et al*, 2003). Long-term follow-up studies have also demonstrated that outcome at two years strongly predicts outcomes 15 years later (Harrison *et al*, 2001). Birchwood *et al* (1998) argue that these observations support the concept that the early phase of psychosis constitutes a 'critical period' in treatment, with major implications for secondary prevention of impairments and disabilities, and provide a further rationale for intervening intensively and early.

Early intervention for psychosis has now become a political priority in the UK and early intervention services (EIS) are being developed across England. The UK Government first announced the intention to develop EIS for young people in 1998. The National Plan for the NHS in 2000 further stated that:

> *Fifty early intervention teams will be established by 2004 so that . . . all young people who experience a first episode of psychosis, such as schizophrenia will receive the early and intensive support they need*

> (Department of Health, 2000, p. 119).

In practice, most GPs see one or two new people with FEP each year. GPs are frequently consulted at some point during a developing FEP, and are the most common final referral agent to EIS in the patient pathway (Skeate *et al*, 2002). GP involvement is also associated with a reduced use of the Mental Health Act (Burnett *et al*, 1999). While FEP is relatively rare from an individual GP's perspective, it is a life-changing event for the person and their family, all of whom often require long-term support and guidance. Primary care therefore has a potentially pivotal role in reducing DUP and influencing the course and outcome of FEP.

Early detection is a challenge for GPs, when psychosis can take several months to emerge from a prodrome of non-specific psychological and social disturbances of varying intensity that can be difficult to distinguish from normal adolescent behaviour. Psychosis rarely presents in neat parcels, and symptoms are rarely volunteered spontaneously. An 'active watching brief' typifies an approach that might regard non-attendance as a signal of deterioration rather than symptom resolution. Such an approach would also involve actively seeking positive and negative psychotic symptoms, and suicidal ideation. Parental fears and intuition should be particularly heeded, and sensitivity given to the impact of an emerging psychosis on the family. GPs should have a high index of suspicion and initially at least, when symptoms are vague, a low threshold for urgently referring a young person with possible FEP for specialist mental health assessment. However by keeping an 'active watching brief', a referral can be made if symptoms persist or become worse. A better GP/patient relationship may well also have been built up, which makes referral less problematic. It is also important to work with the family as therapeutic allies and to be aware of the health needs of the carers themselves. In the longer term, the GP may need to help them obtain information and practical assistance and provide emotional support in coping.

Primary care involvement in FEP is now a part of UK Government strategy, but still relies on GPs acquiring the skills and knowledge to be effective partners in care with both secondary care mental health services and families. A recent survey in Switzerland of 1089 GPs found that their diagnostic and treatment knowledge in FEP was inconsistent, and that only one-third would continue treatment after an FEP, in line with international recommendations (Simon *et al*, 2005). An unpublished study by the author using the same questionnaire with 712 GPs in England found that 95% of GPs have received no recent education on FEP. Most GPs also held pessimistic views about the prognosis of FEP, its early detection and the impact of EIS. There appears, therefore, to be something of a rhetoric/reality gap between policy intentions and consultation-level care. Current work in Birmingham (England) may, however, provide some insight into effective methods for delivering training in this area to GPs (Lester *et al*, 2005a). The REDIRECT trial includes over 80 practices, half of whom have participated in a two-stage educational process consisting of a video featuring role-plays of primary care consultations, GP-led discussion and discussion with EIS users. GPs particularly valued information about symptoms and signs of FEP, particularly negative symptoms, and the opportunity to gain an insight about living with FEP from users themselves. The effect of the training on GPs' abilities to diagnose young people with FEP at an early stage is, however, still being evaluated.

Models of collaborative working

In the UK, there have been a variety of policy initiatives during the last decade that have aimed to increase the role of primary care in the delivery of healthcare to people with SEMI. Primary care, for example, has specific responsibility for delivering standards two and three of the *National Service Framework* (NSF) *for Mental Health* (Department of Health, 1999) and is also integrally involved in the delivery of the other five standards. (The NSF addresses the mental health needs of working age adults up to 65 years. It sets out national standards; national service models; local action and national underpinning programmes for implementation; and a series of national milestones to assure progress, with performance indicators to support effective performance management.) The recent five-year review of the NSF (Department of Health, 2004) also suggests that primary care is seen as the key locus for care for improving mental health services.

Since 1997 and the election of a New Labour Government, there has also been an emphasis on partnership working, with a firm commitment to developing 'joined up solutions' to 'joined up problems'. Work undertaken by the Sainsbury Centre for Mental Health in London suggests that partnership working is a 'must do' in mental health, for a number of political, financial and practical reasons (Sainsbury Centre for Mental Health, 2000). Mental health is complex, with a range of different agencies involved (including healthcare, social care, housing, welfare advice and the employment services). Many patients with SEMI are vulnerable and have limited capacity to negotiate complex bureaucracies. They therefore need services that are well integrated at the point of contact, are easy to negotiate and are focused on their needs. Partnership working can also help to minimise bureaucracy and duplication. Above all, partnership working seems to be beneficial for patients and their carers, who can often experience fragmented services, a lack of continuity of care and conflicting information in situations where local agencies fail to collaborate effectively. This has been described by Preston *et al* (1999) in terms of being 'left in limbo', with users and carers feeling that they are failing to make progress through the healthcare system:

> *Separate clinics don't talk to each other or ring each other. I find the whole thing incredible the length of time it takes; it's just been horrendous, waiting weeks to see a consultant to be told 'I don't know why you've been referred to me' . . . It can make you feel very insignificant*
>
> (patient, quoted in Preston *et al*, 1999, p. 19).

The expansion of 'shared care' schemes between primary care and secondary care (community- and hospital-based services) similarly reflects the importance of partnership working. Models of shared care include 'shifted outpatient clinics', where psychiatrists hold outpatient clinics in primary care surgeries, attaching mental health workers such as CPNs to a primary care surgery rather than basing them in the community, and 'consultation liaison' models, where primary care teams meet up regularly with the local lead psychiatrist to discuss issues and be supported in managing more challenging patients in a primary care setting. Each model of course has its own set of strengths and weaknesses (Lester *et al*, 2004) with no 'ideal' model.

Smaller-scale local, but nevertheless interesting, schemes have also been piloted in the UK to encourage better communication between primary and secondary care services, the rationale being that if roles and responsibilities are clearer and fully documented and communication channels are improved, fewer patients with SEMI will slip between the pavement cracks. Patient-held records, where the person with the medical condition holds all or some information relating to the course and care of their illness, are common in the management of chronic physical illnesses such as diabetes, and have been found to be acceptable to both clinicians and patients with SEMI, and able to improve communication across the primary/secondary care interface (Warner *et al*, 2000; Lester *et al*, 2003a). They do not, however, affect longer-term outcomes such as a reduction in symptoms and satisfaction with care. In London, a Mental Health Link programme has been set up to encourage GPs and associated community mental health teams to work together to develop a series of options for the configuration of shared care for people with SEMI. These include the placement of 'aligned caseload' link workers, guidance on setting up registers, databases and systems of recall, the development of shared care agreements, and an annual joint review of patients' notes to detect and address unmet mental and physical healthcare needs. Evaluation using a cluster randomised controlled trial found significant reductions in relapse rates and increased practitioner satisfaction in the intervention practices, echoing US experiences of integrated care (Byng *et al*, 2004). However, these local schemes, whilst innovative and in many senses successful, had no extra funding attached to them and have not been widely adopted.

The advent and impact of the Quality and Outcomes Framework

Perhaps the biggest sea change in the delivery of primary care for people with SEMI was precipitated by the introduction of a type of performance-related pay into the UK primary healthcare system in April 2004 (British Medical Association (BMA)/NHS Confederation, 2003). The Quality and Outcomes Framework (QOF) is a voluntary mechanism that pays practices for achieving health-related targets across 10 disease areas (and a variety of organisational, patient experience and additional services). There are 1050 points attached to 176 evidence-based indicators, with each point equating to £125.00 that can be earned by the practice on an annual basis. There is an interesting literature on the pros and cons of motivating behaviour change with money, but a clear message from the psychological literature in this area is that incentivising relatively simple tasks will motivate both the financially driven more self-interested 'knave' and the altruistic 'knight' practitioner (Le Grand, 2003).

When initially introduced, there were five indicators in the QOF related to the care of people with SEMI, representing a total of 41 points. The indicators encouraged the development of a register, monitoring of patients on lithium therapy and a review of physical health, medication and co-ordination arrangements with secondary care on an annual basis. Previous attempts at introducing financial incentives in this area of healthcare have led to reviews being carried out but little change in the care or functioning of patients (Kendrick *et al*, 1995). However the combination of an integrated multidisciplinary approach, with registers, integrated IT, training, recall and involvement of patients and elements of the QOF, can bring about a substantial change in care (Wagner, 2000). Practice nurses are, of course, key players in this model of primary care.

It is still far too soon to see if these largely process measures have had an effect on patient health outcomes, but it is encouraging to see that practices across England achieved an average of 89% of the points in the mental health domain. Since the indicators are evidence based, there is every reason to expect positive changes in the morbidity and mortality of people with SEMI over the next decade. Changes in the QOF from April 2006 include fewer points attached to lithium indicators (since these applied to under 30 000 patients in England) and the introduction of two new indicators that encourage GPs to look beyond physical health to wider social issues and which may challenge underlying negative stereotypes of people with SEMI. The first new indicator encourages GPs to document a 'comprehensive care plan' in the primary care record that should include a list of the patient's early warning signs (their illness signature) (Birchwood *et al*, 2000) and discussion of financial benefits and employment opportunities. Discussion of benefits and work may be relatively challenging for some practices, but should also raise awareness within primary care of the social exclusion faced by the majority of people with SEMI. Unemployment rates for this population range from 8% to 20%, with particularly low rates (4% to 12%) for people with schizophrenia (Perkins and Rinaldi, 2002). This new indicator will also complement planned changes to involve primary care more in helping to encourage people back to work as part of the Department for Work and Pensions *Pathways to Work* initiative (Department for Work and Pensions, 2002). The second new indicator requires the practice to actively follow up any patient who has not attended their annual health check, since there is evidence that people who fail to attend may do so because of worsening symptoms rather than a desire to waste a primary care appointment (Lester *et al*, 2005b).

The role of GPs with a special interest

Allied to these changes, which essentially increase the role of primary care in the care of people with SEMI, is a separate UK policy strand that encourages the development of GPs with a special interest (GPwSIs) (Department of Health, 2003a).

GPwSIs in mental health can have a clinical role in

> *providing assessment, advice, information and treatment on behalf of primary care colleagues . . . in most cases working alongside other mental health providers . . . and supporting the development of care pathways across the primary–secondary– community interface*

(Department of Health, 2003a, p. 2).

This new role may provide a mechanism for longer consultations and enable patients to see a GP with a greater knowledge base about mental health issues. It may also encourage more seamless care between primary and secondary care teams. However, by the very nature of being referred on to a GPwSI by their usual GP, continuity of care, which is particularly important for people with SEMI (Crawford *et al*, 2004) may be reduced, opportunities for taking a more holistic individual approach may be missed and the special nature of 'cradle to grave' primary care may be eroded. On a more practical level, there is currently no nationally recognised training programme or accreditation for this role, which has implications from a risk-management perspective. Recent evidence from a randomised controlled trial in the UK of GPwSIs in dermatology has also suggested that although the role may improve access, it may be less cost-effective than usual care (Salisbury *et al*, 2005). Perhaps most importantly, there is also some evidence that patients with SEMI don't necessarily want a specialist in primary care mental health, but may rather have a GP who can provide 'good enough care' (Lester *et al*, 2005b).

The experience of providing and receiving primary care

Listening to what patients want, the 'patient choice agenda', has become an increasingly strong political imperative in the last decade, fuelled by the wider availability of information, treatment options and a slowly growing private sector as well as a more overt recognition of the importance of the concept of consumerism within healthcare. Recently, we have had a new patient tsar and a Command Paper, *Building on the Best* (Department of Health, 2003b) that sets out a series of measures to extend patient choice across primary, secondary and community care. The whole notion of choice, however, is at best a relative concept for people with SEMI, who are subject to compulsory detention, often have no obvious exit from the healthcare system, and are frequently socially excluded.

There has, to date, been relatively little published about the views on primary care of patients with SEMI. Bindman *et al* (1997) found generally high satisfaction scores for primary care services, but mixed patient views on greater GP involvement in shared care. Longitudinal and interpersonal continuity of care, relative ease of access and the option of a home visit are valued features of primary care and often contrasted with the difficulty of seeing a constant stream of new faces in secondary care mental health services. Shared care was perceived by most patients as an 'ideal' state, offering secondary care expertise and primary care continuity. A recent focus group study (Lester *et al*, 2005b) involving groups of GPs and people with SEMI talking together about how to configure good-quality care, found that primary care was seen as the 'cornerstone' of care. Patients clearly prioritised continuity of care, attitudes and willingness to listen and learn over a GP with specialised mental health knowledge. This suggests tensions with the current policy on GPwSIs and also challenges health professionals' assumption that mental health expertise is vital to providing care for patients with SEMI. The views of patients on the importance of personal qualities and attitudes over detailed knowledge also suggest the potential importance of advocacy services in primary care for people with SEMI. This reflects the evidence base on advocacy in the Social Exclusion Unit's report on mental health (Office of the Deputy Prime Minister, 2004), and a recent Rethink survey of 3033 service users that found 28% of people identified greater provision of advocacy as one of their top three priorities for mental health service improvement (Rethink, 2003). This is an area of care where counsellors and members of other professions allied to medicine who may feel their training and clinical experience leave them under-prepared for working with people with SEMI, may have an increasingly important and valuable role to play.

A further interesting aspect of recent work on users' views of primary care emphasises the importance of therapeutic optimism from health professionals, and reflects important underpinning recovery principles of EIS (Warner, 2003). Although many health professionals associate a diagnosis of SEMI with notions of chronicity, patients with SEMI do not necessarily identify themselves as someone living with a *chronic* illness. They prefer a social model of illness that emphasises recovery at least in terms of quality of life issues such as returning to work and regaining family ties (Lester *et al*, 2003b, 2005b).

Conclusion

Mental health policy now recognises the central importance of primary care in the care of people with SEMI. Primary care is a key pathway player at the point of diagnosis, may have a critical role to play in reducing DUP, and has an ongoing role in providing good-quality proactive physical and mental healthcare. However, there is a need for greater training and support for primary care teams to be effective both at the onset and later on in the illness pathway. Secondary care mental health services also need to work in partnership with primary care teams, with clear channels of communication at all stages of the diagnostic and treatment process. The primary care team also needs to remember that they are supporting not just an individual, but also their wider family, as they come to terms with the diagnosis and seek to make sense of the illness.

References

Bindman J, Johnson S, Wright S *et al* (1997) Integration between primary and secondary services in the care of the severely mentally ill: patients' and general practitioners' views. *British Journal of Psychiatry* 171:169–74.

Birchwood M, Spencer E and McGovern D (2000) Schizophrenia: early warning signs. *Advances in Psychiatric Treatment* 6:93–101.

Birchwood M, Todd P and Jackson C (1998) Early intervention in psychosis, the critical period hypothesis. *British Journal of Psychiatry* 172(Suppl. 33):53–9.

Bird L (1999) *The Fundamental Facts about Mental Illness.* London: Mental Health Foundation.

BMA/NHS Confederation (2003) *Investing in General Practice: the new general medical services contract.* London: BMA.

Brown J, Weich S, Downes-Grainger E and Goldberg D (1999a) Attitudes of inner city GPs to shared care for psychiatric patients in the community. *British Journal of General Practice* 49:643–4.

Brown S, Birtwhistle J, Roe L and Thompson C (1999b) The unhealthy lifestyle of people with schizophrenia. *Psychological Medicine* 29:697–701.

Burnett R, Mallett R, Bhugra G *et al.* (1999) The first contact of patients with schizophrenia with psychiatric services: social factors and pathways to care in a multi-ethnic population. *Psychological Medicine* 29:475–83.

Burns T and Cohen A (1998) Item-of-service payments for GP care of severely mentally ill persons. *British Journal of General Practice* 48:1415–16.

Burns T, Greenwood N, Kendrick T and Garland C (2000) Attitudes of general practitioners and community mental health team staff towards the locus of care for people with chronic psychotic disorders. *Primary Care Psychiatry* 6:67–71.

Byng R, Jones R, Leese M *et al* (2004) Exploratory cluster randomised controlled trial of shared care development for long-term mental illness. *British Journal of General Practice* 54:259–66.

Chong SA, Mythily S and Mahendran R (2001) Cardiac effects of psychotropic drugs. *Annals of the Academy of Medicine of Singapore* 30:625–31.

Connolly M and Kelly C (2005) Lifestyle and physical health in schizophrenia. *Advances in Psychiatric Treatment* 11:125–32.

Crawford MJ, de Jonge E, Freeman GK and Weaver T (2004) Providing continuity of care for people with severe mental illness – a narrative review. *Social Psychiatry and Psychiatric Epidemiology* 39:265–72.

Crosland A and Kai J (1998) They think they can talk to nurses: practice nurses' views of their roles in caring for mental health problems. *British Journal of General Practice* 48:1383–6.

Department of Health (1999) *The National Service Framework for Mental Health.* London: Department of Health.

Department of Health (2000) *The NHS Plan: a plan for investment, a plan for reform.* London: Department of Health.

Department of Health (2003a) *Guidelines for the Appointment of General Practitioners with Special Interests in the Delivery of Clinical Services: mental health.* London: Department of Health.

Department of Health (2003b) *Building on the Best: choice, responsiveness and equity in the NHS.* London: The Stationery Office.

Department of Health (2004) *The National Service Framework for Mental Health – Five Years on.* London: Department of Health.

Department for Work and Pensions (2002) *Pathways to Work: helping people into employment*. London: The Stationery Office. www.dwp.gov.uk/consultations/consult/2002/pathways/pathways.pdf (accessed 3 January 2007).

Disability Rights Commission (2005) *Equal Treatment: closing the gap*. London: Disability Rights Commission.

Gray R, Parr AM, Plummer S *et al* (1999) A national survey of practice nurse involvement in mental health interventions. *Journal of Advanced Nursing* 30:901–6.

Harrigan SM, McGorry PD and Krstev H (2003) Does treatment delay in first-episode psychosis really matter? *Psychological Medicine* 33:97–110.

Harris EC and Barraclough B (1998) Excess mortality of mental disorder. *British Journal of Psychiatry* 173:11–53.

Harrison G, Hopper K, Craig T *et al* (2001) Recovery from psychotic illness: a 15 and 25 year international follow up study. *British Journal of Psychiatry* 178:506–17.

Jenkins R, McCulloch A, Friedli L and Park C (2002) *Developing a National Mental Health Policy*. London: Maudsley Monograph.

Kai J, Crosland A and Drinkwater C (2000) Prevalence of enduring and disabling mental illness in the inner city. *British Journal of General Practice* 50:922–4.

Kendrick T (1996) Cardiovascular and respiratory risk factors and symptoms among general practice patients with long-term mental illness. *British Journal of Psychiatry* 169: 733–9.

Kendrick T, Burns T and Freeling P (1995) Randomised controlled trial of general practitioners to carry out structured assessments of their long term mentally ill patients. *British Medical Journal* 311:93–8.

Kendrick T, Sibbald B, Burns T and Freeling P (1991) Role of general practitioners in care of long term mentally ill patients. *British Medical Journal* 302:508–10.

Lang F, Johnstone E and Murray D (1997) Service provision for people with schizophrenia. Role of the general practitioner. *British Journal of Psychiatry* 171:165–8.

Lawrie SM, Martin K, McNeill G *et al* (1998) General practitioners' attitudes to psychiatric and medical illness. *Psychological Medicine* 28:1463–7.

Lawrie SM, Parsons C, Patrick J *et al* (1996) A controlled trial of general practitioners' attitudes to patients with schizophrenia. *Health Bulletin* 54:210–13.

Le Grand J (2003) *Motivation, Agency and Public Policy: of knight and knaves, pawns and queens*. Oxford: Oxford University Press.

Lester HE, Glasby J and Tylee A (2004) Integrated primary care mental health: threat or opportunity in the new NHS? *British Journal of General Practice* 54:282–91.

Lester H, Jowett S, Wilson S, Allan T and Roberts L (2003a) A cluster randomised controlled trial of patient medical records for people with schizophrenia receiving shared care. *British Journal of General Practice* 53:197–203.

Lester HE, Tait L, Khera A and Birchwood M (2005a) The development and evaluation of an educational intervention on first episode psychosis for primary care. *Medical Education* 39:1006–14.

Lester HE, Tritter J and England E (2003b) Satisfaction with primary care: the perspectives of people with schizophrenia. *Family Practice* 20:508–13.

Lester HE, Tritter JQ and Sorohan H (2005b) Providing primary care for people with serious mental illness: a focus group study. *British Medical Journal* 330:1122–8.

McGlashan TH (1999) Duration of untreated psychosis in first episode schizophrenia: Marker or determinant of course. *Biological Psychiatry* 46:899–907.

Mental After Care Association (1999) *First National GP Survey of Mental Health in Primary Care*. London: Mental After Care Association.

Miller J (1991) *Openmind* 49:6–7.

Mukherjee S, Decina P, Bocola V *et al* (1996) Diabetes mellitus in schizophrenic patients. *Comprehensive Psychiatry* 37:68–73.

Nazareth I, King M, Haines A *et al* (1993) Care of schizophrenia in general practice. *British Medical Journal* 307:910.

Office of the Deputy Prime Minister (2004) *Mental Health and Social Exclusion (Social Exclusion Unit Report)*. London: Office of the Deputy Prime Minister.

Oyesanmi O, Kunkel EJ, Monti DA *et al* (1999) Hematologic side effects of psychotropics. *Psychosomatics* 40:414–21.

Perkins R and Rinaldi M (2002) Unemployment rates among patients with long-term mental health problems. *Psychiatric Bulletin* 26:295–8.

Preston C, Cheater F, Baker R and Hearnshaw H (1999) Left in limbo: patients' views on care across the primary/secondary interface. *Quality in Health Care* 8:16–21.

Rethink (2003) *Just One Per Cent*. London: Rethink.

Sainsbury Centre for Mental Health (2000) *Taking your partners: using opportunities for inter-agency partnership in mental health*. London: Sainsbury Centre for Mental Health.

Salisbury C, Noble A, Horrocks S *et al* (2005) Evaluation of a GPSI services for dermatology: a randomised controlled trial. *British Medical Journal* 331:1441–6.

Sernyak MJ, Leslie DL, Alarcon RD, Losonczy MF and Rosenheck R (2002) Association of diabetes mellitus with use of atypical neuroleptics in the treatment of schizophrenia. *American Journal of Psychiatry* 159:561–6.

Simon A, Lauber C, Ludewig K *et al* (2005) General practitioners and schizophrenia: results from a Swiss survey. *British Journal of Psychiatry* 187:274–81.

Singleton N, Bumpstead R, O'Brien M, Lee A and Meltzer H (2001) *Psychiatric Morbidity Among Adults Living in Private Households, 2000*. London: The Stationery Office.

Skeate A, Jackson C, Birchwood M and Jones C (2002) Duration of untreated psychosis and pathways to care in first-episode psychosis. *British Journal of Psychiatry* 181:s73–7.

Wagner EH (2000) The role of patient care teams in chronic disease management. *British Medical Journal* 320:569–72.

Warner JP, King M, Blizard R, McClenahan Z and Tang S (2000) Patient-held shared care records for individuals with mental illness. *British Journal of Psychiatry* 177:319–24.

Warner R (2003) *Recovery from Schizophrenia: psychiatry and political economy* (3e). Hove and New York: Brunner-Routledge.

Chapter 5

Filling the gap: creating models of care for people with long-term, complex, non-psychotic mental health problems

Richard Byng

Introduction

The literature on primary care mental health has tended to focus on those with common mental health problems and those with psychosis, including bipolar disorder. This leads to the impression that most common mental health problems are new onset, whereas as many as 60% are recurrent (Vuorilehto *et al*, 2005). Depression and other problems are beginning to be seen as long-term, chronic diseases (Andrews, 2001), and although this is not always the case, systems of individual and organisational care need to take this into account. Within an individual practice there are many more people with disability resulting from long-term non-psychotic illnesses than there are those with psychosis. The burden is, as a result, of considerable co-morbidity (Andrews *et al*, 1998). The effects are profound on the individual, but also are significant when considering family members, particularly children, and the economy as a whole. This chapter will outline different ways of defining this complex group, consider deficits in care, and propose ways in which individual care and the organisation of care can be enhanced, using a combination of inferences from the literature, case studies, personal experience and predictions.

Defining the population

There are several ways in which to define the population to which I am referring. This section will outline both the traditional epidemiological and medical definition based on DSM or ICD diagnoses, but will also examine other more pragmatic ways of identifying the population, such as medication use on general practice databases.

Chronic and recurrent depression are probably the most important diagnostic descriptors because of their prevalence and impact. People with long-term depression (LTD) lie along spectra of severity and recurrence rates. This chapter adopts a pragmatic definition suitable for primary care, including recurrent major depression (three or more episodes) and chronic depression (lasting more than two years). The spectra include those with recurrent brief episodes of moderate depression, through to those with severe and enduring disability (Andrews,

2001). The majority of those diagnosed with depression have a history of recurrent depression. There is a wide range of co-morbidities associated with LTD including: chronic physical conditions; diagnoses such as general anxiety disorder, panic and post-traumatic stress disorder (PTSD); personality disorders and drug and alcohol problems. Only 12% of those with LTD have no co-morbidity (Vuorilehto *et al*, 2005). Ongoing mental illness is associated with social disadvantage, either as a cause of or as a result of the mental health problem (Rogers and Pilgrim, 2003). Only 26% of those disabled due to depression and other long-term neurotic conditions are in work, compared with a mean of 50% for all causes of disability (Office for National Statistics, 2005).

Those with ongoing problems such as chronic anxiety and other conditions such as PTSD, obsessive–compulsive disorder (OCD) and panic disorder nearly always have some degree of recurrent or chronic depression as a result, but if they do not they are also included in the 'three Ds definition' (Slade *et al*, 1997, *see* Box 5.1). Similarly those with chronic substance misuse problems often have recurrent or chronic depression. Those with a history of anorexia and eating disorders often go on to have recurrent depression. Many of these people can also be classified as having personality disorders, and many with significant personality disorders also have depression or other diagnoses, although a significant proportion of those with borderline and histrionic personality disorders do not meet the criteria for depression. While there is debate about the value of personality-based diagnoses, the descriptions of thoughts and behaviours associated with these persistent problems are useful for assessing needs for treatment and care.

The 'three Ds definition' is useful for primary and community care because of its emphasis on significant but less severe disability. This requires a *diagnosis* of some kind, a *duration* of two or more years and ongoing *disability*, as defined in Box 5.1. It clearly moves the agenda on from the false 'psychosis–common mental health problem' dichotomy, and brings in social functioning as a means of defining the problem. This opens up possibilities for outcome-based care, with social inclusion as a desired end-point.

Box 5.1   Three Ds Model: inclusion criteria for long-term mental illness

Diagnosis

Patients having:

- *either*: one of the *psychoses*, including schizophrenia, paranoid psychosis, manic-depressive psychosis and psychotic depression (excluding those with no medication and no episode/care needs for 3 years)
- *or*: one of the *chronic non-psychotic* disorders with a substantial *disability and a duration of two years or more*, for example: recurrent or continuing major depression, severe anxiety, panic and phobic disorders, OCD and PTSD.

Duration

The patient's disability must have been present for two years or more, including frequent recurrences or stable problems requiring ongoing medication or support.

Disability

Disability may be defined as being unable to fulfil any one of the following:
- being able to hold down a job
- maintaining self-care and personal hygiene
- performing necessary domestic chores
- participating in recreational activities

The disability must be due to any one or more of four types of impairment of social behaviour:
- withdrawal and inactivity
- avoidance behaviour
- bizarre or embarrassing behaviour
- violence towards others or self.

Epidemiology

The prevalence of severe and enduring non-psychotic conditions varied from 1.3 to 8.3/1000 in recent studies (Kendrick et al, 1994; Kai et al, 2000). Long-term antidepressant prescribing is an additional and convenient marker in primary care; in one practice, 36 per 1000 of the population were on long-term psychotropic medication, predominantly anxiolytics and antidepressants, and these patients were markedly more distressed than controls (Catalan et al, 1988). There are no recent UK studies examining prevalence and need. In the US, 75% of primary care-treated patients reported ongoing depression (Schwenk et al, 2004). So, while not all those on long-term antidepressants would reach criteria for LTD, all would have care needs: those in remission from recurrence will merit preventive management; some will need support in overcoming fears to come off antidepressants; others will be in partial remission or an ongoing episode, and will need assertive management to address depression and other physical and mental health conditions.

Improving care

Several components of care are necessary for managing chronic disease (Wagner, 1998). These include patient involvement (including self-help), collaboration with specialist services, an appropriate review function and service redesign to incorporate these features. Reviewing care in particular is associated with better outcomes for depression (Von Korff and Goldberg, 2001). Medication combined with psychosocial modalities has been shown to improve outcomes (Arnow and Constantino, 2003). Currently, primary care, with its mainly reactive response, and secondary care, with its emphasis on psychosis, are not fulfilling the needs of those with chronic and relapsing depression and other ongoing non-psychotic conditions; voluntary sector organisations have poor links with primary care, but have the potential to provide collaboration. Although facilitated self-help is being developed for more time-limited mental health problems, patient involvement has not been well developed for LTD. The use of recovery-based models, relapse recognition, self-help groups and facilitated self-help all require evaluation for people with LTD.

Care for individuals

This section will outline how primary care teams can be involved in the care of people with complex, non-psychotic conditions over a number of months and years. The lynchpin for this provision will often be the primary care practitioner, often a GP, but perhaps an experienced nurse or counsellor, and, in the future, we might see specialist mental health workers taking a lead. Having a named primary care worker addresses a major issue for many patients – continuity. This practitioner can then juggle, organise and co-ordinate various modalities, including the psychological, the medical and the social. These modalities will need to be introduced within an overall framework which is safe, involves an exchange of views, fully engages the individual concerned, and offers choice and involvement in decision making at all levels.

The medical paradigm

The medical perspective is important in terms of managing an analysis of the problem with respect to diagnosis, assessing risk and providing medical treatments. Many people with long-term mental health problems feel stigmatised and may find it difficult to engage with practitioners in primary care. They may not recognise that they have mental health problems, being more concerned abut co-morbid physical health issues. A trusting relationship that addresses the need for ongoing care must first involve an explicit discussion about psychological distress and, if possible, a discussion about the diagnosis. Practitioners need to ensure that a range of specific psychiatric diagnoses are not missed. For example, those with chronic depression will need to have specific screening questions asked, e.g. about feeling the need to do things in certain ways, recurring thoughts and dreams about traumatic events to ensure that they don't also have disorders such as OCD, PTSD, panic or eating disorders. Alcohol and drug addictions and problems such as bipolar affective disorder and other psychoses should also be excluded. Screening for personality problems is less well developed within the primary care setting. The aim of these questions is not so much to classify as to identify specific problems or issues that may be amenable to particular medications or psychological treatment strategies.

Medication is likely to continue to play a considerable role in the management of people with these long-term problems. Occasionally, in times of great distress benzodiazepines and other hypnotics or anxiolytics may be useful. While these have been shown to have effectiveness in the short term, the addictive qualities of these medications will often outweigh their introduction even for short-term treatment. They may also result in a sense of disempowerment and belief that only these particular medications will improve wellbeing. *See* Freeth (2004) for a full discussion on the relevant medication.

Psychological work

Practitioners caring for this group of patients will also benefit from some knowledge of psychological therapies and their theoretical orientations. As a minimum they should have an understanding of the difference between approaches such as Rogerian counselling, cognitive-behavioural approaches, psychodynamic approaches and psychoanalysis. Many people, both patients and practitioners, will want to know more about a range of other treatment options. In reality, at the moment, knowledge and understanding of these treatment modalities are restricted by lack of availability. Psychological therapy for this group of patients may be appropriate at the time of greatest distress during relapse or recurrence, but also may be relevant during periods of recovery as a buffer against further relapses. For example, CBT has now been shown to be as effective as antidepressants, and additive to medication in the prevention of further episodes of depression for those with recurrence. A range of other psychological treatments, outlined more fully in other chapters of this book, may well be relevant as part of a recovery and relapse-prevention plan for those who have come out of the depths of crisis. The GP's role will often be to discuss the possibility of various modalities, including whether it is a one-to-one approach or group work, whether there is a long or short waiting list, whether it is a short-term or long-term treatment package, or whether it involves interfacing with a computer or book, rather than a therapist. The GP–nurse–counsellor triangle can be a very supportive team, helpful for patients and practitioners alike. This discussion and triage function is important, and if the generalist practitioner has insufficient knowledge then it may well be carried out by an experienced counsellor, psychotherapist or specialist mental health practitioner. Those practices with experienced link workers or a generic counselling, psychotherapy or psychological therapy team that carries out assessments may be able to provide or refer to such services. Where in-house generic counselling, psychotherapy or psychological therapy exists in the practice, it will most likely be appropriate to refer for a first treatment/assessment with an experienced counsellor, psychologist or psychotherapist. This is a convincing argument for counselling and psychotherapy courses to include mental health as a 'must' on all levels of training.

It is also important not to underestimate the psychological role of the generic practitioner. Some GPs and other primary healthcare team (PHCT) members will have undergone training in counselling, cognitive-behavioural or solution-focused therapy, so that these approaches can be integrated within consultations. However, every practitioner has a role in listening, providing empathy and validating a patient's narrative (Launer, 2002).

Health-promoting opportunities and social interventions

Mental health promotion is an important means of keeping people well. It is very important for those with long-term mental health problems. Patients believe that social contact, walking the dog and fresh air are important means of recovery, and there are indeed potentially effective underlying mechanisms for these beliefs (Lauber *et al*, 2001). Exercise has now been proven to be effective for those with depression, and there is increasing evidence to support healthy diets to promote mental health (Craft and Landers, 1998). Often advice and encouragement towards a more healthy lifestyle involve an understanding of the individual's preferences and social situation and a discussion about the balance between work and leisure; sleep, rest and activity; relaxation and stimulation and interaction with others alongside time to reflect alone. Individuals may well know the pathway that is best for them, but might benefit from a structured review of these issues to reflect on.

An understanding of the individual's social context both contributes to defining the level of illness and also points the way towards recovery. This might include assessment of their work situation, their leisure activities, their housing, the number of social contacts they have, their family situation, their interest in exercise and sport and their involvement in religious or spiritual activities. People with longstanding mental health problems often participate less in these areas. Possibly the most critical of these is employment, which so defines our status. While in some inner-city areas unemployment is no longer a stigma, for most people lack of work, or lack of engagement in productive or creative activity is a continuing source of demoralisation. While some people are genuinely caught in benefits traps and are unable to move easily into paid employment, most will be able to identify creative experiences that they have enjoyed or would like to engage in. Practitioners can help facilitate involvement in opportunities within their locality.

Recent pilots have shown that supporting people in long-term unemployment back to work has benefits in terms of both the individual's finances and their mental state. Counsellors and psychotherapists can play a large role in supporting their clients through such times of transition. New legislation on incapacity benefit and support to help people to return to work is likely to provide many opportunities for primary care workers to support individuals back to work.

Others are too unwell to return to work and many require very practical support, such as to obtain benefits, while other may simply need to be listened to or be in counselling/psychotherapy. Volunteering opportunities are also on offer. Volunteering in a small way can be both a step towards paid employment and a useful activity in itself. Limited hours of volunteering are allowable under the benefits system. It is likely that the new pathways to work legislation will encourage volunteering as one of the paths back to paid employment. Currently, unfortunately, there are few organisations that combine advice on benefits, volunteering and employment.

'Time banks' are a particular form of volunteering where individuals join an organisation and swap resources and favours. Box 5.2 shows the example of a case study in South East London, where a time bank based in a practice was able to provide opportunities for individuals with a variety of mental health problems to gain confidence and feel empowered through doing rather than receiving.

Box 5.2   Time heals! London practice helps patients heal themselves – by using time as a currency

The Rushey Green Group Practice in Catford can now prescribe time for those who are depressed, lonely, feel disempowered or just want to meet others and have some fun. The time bank is like a club within the practice where members meet, work together and swap favours.

The concept of 'time dollars' and 'time banks' was developed by Dr Edgar Cahn as a way of introducing non-medical services for older people – helping them to stay in their own homes, keep hospital appointments and stay healthy.

Time banks are one way of putting neighbours in touch with each other, using people's skills and imagination, particularly older people's, which are often ignored, and building a network of neighbourhood support. They are co-ordinated by a paid time broker, who recruits members, links up people who can help each other, and records transactions in the free 'TimeKeeper' software. One hour shared equals one time credit.

Edgar Cahn visited the Rushey Green Health Centre to talk to GPs, health workers and patients about how the time bank could make a difference. The practice worked with the New Economics Foundation to develop the idea, and funding was given to pilot the project by the King's Fund. The Rushey Green time bank was launched in March 2000.

The Rushey Green time bank has between 80 and 100 members at any time including several organisations. The range and type of services include: befriending, running errands, giving lifts, arranging social events, woodwork, poetry writing, babysitting, gardening, swimming, fishing, teaching the piano, catering, and giving local knowledge.

Many members are from minority ethnic groups, about one-third are over 65 years old, and half have some kind of disability, most with a mental health component. This focus on the elderly and disabled has meant additional work compared with other non-health-based time banks. The bank has now become an integral part of the practice, but has also become self-running, with charitable status and an independent constitution.

GPs and health workers at the practice make most of the referrals; others come from members recruiting in the waiting rooms and amongst neighbours, and from outside agencies.

A survey of time bank members found that the time bank had:

- improved participants' social networks outside of their home and family
- given a sense of self-worth to people who had previously been passive recipients of care, and had reduced the burden on traditional carers in the form of both family and social services
- provided an alternative to traditional medical treatments such as antidepressants, for health workers who understand the social causes of ill-health.

For more information on the Rushey Green time bank visit www.london timebank.org.uk or email info@londontimebank.org.uk.

Ensuring continuity and a strategy towards social inclusion

This range of possibilities for people with long-term mental health problems is the basis for ongoing commitment by primary care practitioners to support people with mental health problems in times of crisis and recovery. It requires, if possible, continuity with an allocated primary care worker for each person identified as having long-term mental health problems. This is increasingly important as PHCTs continue to grow in size. Each consultation requires empathy, real listening and shared decision making about the next steps. The use of solution-focused approaches within consultations, building on positive achievements in times of recovery and what the individual is doing to help themselves in times of crisis can empower individuals by emphasising strengths. This will help counter negative feelings about psychological dependence arising from the sole use of medications.

Cognitive-behavioural techniques with staged approaches to achievements can also provide a useful framework for broadening the range of activities in which an individual is engaged. These approaches can help shift people's lives to becoming more included in mainstream activities. The 'inclusion web' is a useful tool that practitioners can use to identify and reflect on domains of life in terms of places frequented and contact with people. It can be used over a series of consultations to map out an individual's life, and identify areas in which they would like to be more involved. This range of strategies and tools to bring together a series of trials of individual treatments for the individual person provides the basis for optimistic practitioners – both generic primary care and specialist mental health.

Developing systems for treatment and recovery

In order to ensure the individual care detailed above can occur, a number of systems within the health services and beyond are important to consider. Within the PHCT there may be adjustments to roles and procedures; individuals need to be fully involved in their care, which will require the development of information systems and new ways of working; specialist input has been shown to improve outcomes and there are a number of different ways in which this may occur; redesigning the systems of care and, in particular, systems to review care will be critical in improving primary care-based services.

Involving individuals in their own care

Providing information and involving individuals in their own care are two facets identified by Wagner *et al* (1996)as being crucial for chronic disease management. When these are applied to people with long-term mental health problems, a number of opportunities might be considered, from those that are focused on information through to those setting up systems for shared decision making and user-led care.

Information is crucial to decision making and the following systems are likely to be required within primary care settings:

- a full set of leaflets about a variety of conditions and treatments
- an up-to-date website available to practitioners and users, detailing all of the local opportunities for care provision
- a website with detailed information at a national level about conditions and treatments, with links to other websites
- a full range of books and details of opportunities at local libraries and other public venues
- information about ways in which people can be involved in their own care and in developing systems of care (e.g. 'wellness recovery action plan' (WRAP, *see* below), inclusion web and 'patients as teachers' organisations).

A number of initiatives provide positive examples of how patients can be involved in their own care. The Rushey Green Time Bank, as outlined in Box 5.2, is an example of how contributing to others can promote mental health. A belief in oneself, or a sense of mastery might be achieved through the experience of being a doer or giver rather than a recipient.

Perhaps the most important range of initiatives for which there is currently growing support is that of patient-led recovery tools. One particular example is the 'wellness recovery action plan' (WRAP) (Copeland, 2005). This is a system of care defined by users to identify ways to help themselves towards recovery and inclusion in social activities; it also details plans for relapses and crisis. Currently these tools are little used in primary care. However, there is no reason why the techniques, principles or simplified versions of the original tools should not be used across a series of primary care consultations.

The Expert Patient Programme has not been fully developed in mental health, but there are examples of how this policy could be utilised. The 'patients as teachers' initiative in Lewisham involved people with depression carrying out research on others with depression, in order to formulate clear guidance on improvements to local care. This provides a model for how they can become involved in local research and evaluation of services, as well as teachers teaching the professionals and students (Patients as Teachers Research Team, 2003).

Expert patients could take on the following roles in a voluntary or paid capacity:

- teaching students and professionals
- helping evaluate and plan services
- providing advocacy and signposting
- running patient support groups.

Systems of review

In the literature of collaborative care for depression coming from the US, systems of review, alongside specialist input have the most evidence as mechanisms for improving outcomes (Von Korff and Goldberg, 2001). Primary care in the UK is based mainly on reactive care, and although the 1991 and 2004 contract revisions have 'incentivised' the use of systems care for chronic disease management, these have been largely confined to physical conditions, and the small incentives for reviewing mental healthcare are now restricted to those with psychosis and bipolar affective disorder. It is therefore urgent that incentives are introduced to ensure the review of people with chronic and recurrent disabling common mental health problems.

The current basis for such review is the repeat-prescribing medication reviews which are carried out well within some practices. However, these rarely involve a systematic assessment of patients' needs in terms of diagnosis, social inclusion, medication and the range of psychosocial interventions that may be appropriate. A small proportion of those with long-term disabling mental health conditions under specialist services will, hopefully, receive ongoing care, and there should be robust systems in place to ensure that patients do not drop out of care. However, with the imperative to move towards a more user-centred care, there is a tension between the 'register and recall' system and ensuring that patients take responsibility for their ongoing management.

An exemplary service might ensure that those flagged as having a long-term, disabling mental health condition should be called for a review once a year at a minimum. For those who are being followed up regularly, this may involve just ensuring that areas not covered during the year are addressed, while for those who have not been seeking care during the year, it would provide an opportunity to systematically address a range of psychological, medication and social issues. For some people this might be carried out by the GP or a named primary care worker, while in some practices and for some patients it might be more appropriate for the graduate mental health worker or linked worker from the CMHT, or indeed a counsellor or psychologist to review psychosocial needs in more detail. If less-experienced workers are used, high-volume supervision may be an effective means of ensuring quality.

Telephone recall has also been used to ensure that those with mental health problems adhere to treatment and maintain contact with services. It has been found to be particularly popular with patients, and effective at improving outcomes in the treatment of acute episodes of common mental health problems and as part of a collaborative care arrangement for those with recurrent depression. This might be run by receptionists or counsellors, given additional training; but could also involve practice nurses or, indeed, GPs making calls.

Whatever the system chosen, there needs to be a named person responsible for chasing those who are not attending, and ensuring that no one is missed from the system. General practices have been particularly effective at ensuring this process occurs for those patients whose follow-up is rewarded in the QOF, and are quite capable of running a system for long-term chronic depression and other conditions.

Development of the primary healthcare team

Primary care teams are dominated in their decision making and process of care by GPs, who have overlapping roles and close links with practice nurses, district nurses, health visitors and practice counsellors. Each of the three community-based nursing roles involves dealing with people with long-term mental health problems. District nurses are often dealing with housebound elderly who invariably have some kind of mental health problems, often depression and anxiety, and suffer from bereavements and loneliness. Health visitors have contact with young mothers, many of whom have mental health problems, and also have responsibility for the mental health of children who may well be affected by parents' mental health problems. Practice nurses come into contact with a wide range of the population whom they might screen for mental health problems but, perhaps more importantly, might be identifying mental health problems in those with long-term physical health conditions. This role is now rewarded within the QOF, and will enhance the role of PHCTs as promoters of both physical and mental wellbeing. Despite this contact with mental health problems, the training of practice nurses in mental health, unless they have undergone registered mental nurse (RMN) training, is often extremely limited. There are few requirements for ongoing postgraduate training, and the nurses themselves are divided between those who want to take on a more psychosocial role and those whose main interest is with physical health. Education in the form of external training, in-house training, supervision and mentoring will be required as these nurses are asked to adapt to a more psychosocial way of thinking and fit into new systems of review and assessment for those with long-term mental health problems. Once community-based nurses gain experience of mental health problems, they are able to go on to take a lead role in the management of ongoing mental healthcare.

Receptionists, as the first point of contact within the PHCT, are another underused resource with respect to mental health and wellbeing. They have very little training in relation to mental health and understanding about how valuable their role could be. When our practice was creating a system to alert receptionists about angry or aggressive patients, it soon became clear that people with depression and other mental health problems were being labelled as 'difficult' by the administrative team. A recent initiative, as part of the Lewisham Depression Programme, has involved the training of receptionists (Clinical Governance Resource Group, 2004). This training has covered recognition of mental health problems, understanding when the receptionist should consider informing a clinical member of staff about a possible mental health problem, and working with practice managers to ensure that job descriptions and team roles of receptionists facilitate identification and ongoing care of people with mental health problems.

Counsellors and psychologists attached to practices may be independent practitioners or employed by primary care trusts or mental health trusts, and very occasionally by GPs themselves. The normal relationship between GPs and counsellors, however, appears to be similar across organisations and consists of referral of individual patients. There may be variable feedback from counsellors depending on their views about confidentiality, and very little liaison work. Some practices have developed liaison models for counsellors and psychologists on a number of different levels. This liaison could consist of a discussion about individual cases when considering referral, meeting monthly or three-monthly at practice meetings to discuss general issues or specific cases. Some practices have developed models where counsellors and psychologists provide consultancy to GPs and practice nurses who are seeing clients on an ongoing basis, with supervision from the counsellor or psychologist.

The role of practice counsellors and psychologists in the care of people with longer-term serious mental illness is disputed. Some counsellors prefer not to become involved in supporting those with more severe disability and depression. My experience is that these rules, based on diagnosis, tend to be unhelpful and that it is more useful to examine the emotional, psychological, and counselling support needs of the individual rather than their past psychiatric history when deciding whether a referral is appropriate. For example, someone with a long history of OCD and depression may well benefit from a period of counselling to address an issue that is related to, but not central to, these diagnoses.

Graduate mental health workers are a new element to the primary care workforce, and primarily work with those with mild to moderate conditions. They are often trained to provide psychological treatment in brief form and to link this to psychosocial interventions. Their lack of experience to date has led their roles to be restricted to dealing mainly with those with new episodes and simple conditions. However, in some areas graduate workers have been specifically asked to provide reports on individuals with more chronic problems. Such documents would generally involve assessing both their psychological and social needs.

Given the dearth of resources for people with longstanding mental health problems, counsellors, psychologists, link workers and graduate mental health workers may all have roles when designing services at practice or locality level. In East Devon the role of a new worker is being designed to fulfil an intermediate position between CMHT-based CPNs and graduate mental health workers and counsellors. Their role will include reviewing those discharged from CMHTs, but also assessing those with chronic problems referred on from GPs whom the community mental health teams would not accept, based on the referral criteria.

Liaison with the voluntary sector

Most areas have significant small and medium-sized voluntary sector organisations. Branches of organisations such as MIND and Depression Alliance exist in most major conurbations. In addition, there are small voluntary sector organisations that have arisen as support groups, for carers or for individual patients, and others that have arisen out of the principles of community development. They often offer patient-centred services which are based on principles of social inclusion but are frequently poorly funded. Funding is often renewed on an annual basis, making planning for expansion difficult. Relationships between primary care and these voluntary sector organisations are normally patchy, with GPs being unaware of these organisations as local resources. Graduate mental health workers and some counsellors have included in their role the identification and formation of links with these organisations to primary care settings. Voluntary sector organisations can play a valuable role in assisting people with benefits advice, advice on voluntary work or perhaps provision of voluntary work plus assisting in pathways to work. They may well work through a number of mechanisms including increasing contact with others and increasing trusting relationships and networks, as well as promoting physical and mental activity. Links between general practices and these organisations can be enhanced by meeting face to face at local events or attendance at practice meetings. Systematic information about these resources should be available from local information systems. This should include clear information about referral criteria, work undertaken, locality, opening times and contact details.

Liaison between primary care and specialist mental health workers and teams

During the 1970s and 1980s, liaison between psychiatrists and GPs developed (Mitchell, 1985). This varied regionally: by the mid-1980s, 50% of Scottish GPs reported an attachment with a psychiatrist (Pullen and Yellowlees, 1988) and in England almost 20% of consultant psychiatrists described spending time in general practice (Strathdee and Williams, 1984). In a parallel development, CPNs were being attached to practices, so that by 1990 50% of practices had CPN attachments (Thomas and Corney, 1992).

However, the form of this liaison was hotly debated. Mitchell (1985) suggested four key elements were required: regular face-to-face contact achieving a mutual understanding, an acceptable meeting place, open communication, and mutual trust. GPs wanted better communication, assessments by specialists in primary care, and to retain responsibility (Strathdee, 1988). The shifted outpatient model was the norm but liaison between the GP and the specialists, either after the consultation or during a shared consultation, was also common (Creed and Marks, 1989). A more a structured version of the liaison model ensured all possible referrals were seen and always discussed afterwards (Gask *et al*, 1997).

These models evolved without a policy imperative and were rarely well evaluated. Williams and Balestrieri (1989) showed that admissions were reduced in areas with a high degree of liaison work. Most evaluations, however, focused on the process and the increased access to specialist care brought about by liaison; there was also increasing concern that attached mental health workers, as well as the new community mental health centres, left those with psychosis with reduced provision (Sayce *et al*, 1991).

A number of high-profile disasters catalysed a policy focus on specialist care for those with psychosis (Ritchie *et al*, 1994). The care programme approach (CPA) and multidisciplinary CMHTs were the mechanisms of implementation (Department of Health, 1994). By the mid-1990s, only fundholding GPs retained linked CPNs and psychiatrists, mostly in the form of 'shifted outpatients' with little liaison. Despite guidance on shared care from the Joint Royal College Working Group (1993), PHCTs and CMHTs developed independently.

Large volumes of referrals from primary care to CMHTs were countered by the development of strict referral criteria for entry to specialist care. This led to deteriorating relationships between primary and secondary care. GPs recognised that patients with psychosis had better care in the reorganised services, but patients with non-psychotic illness were worse off (Harrison *et al*, 1997). GPs generally had low involvement and low satisfaction with the care responsibilities for patients under specialist services (Bindman *et al*, 1997).

To resolve these problems, link workers providing communication between CMHTs and PHCTs were advocated. However, there was rarely an expectation that link workers would preferentially receive referrals from the practices they were linked to. On the other hand Goldberg and Gournay's model was explicit about the need for CPNs to receive referrals from the practices to which they were linked (Goldberg and Gournay, 1997).

Since then, government policy has continued to concentrate on patients with severe mental illness and the establishment of specialised functional teams. Guidance has been much less definitive about liaison between community mental health services and PHCTs. In particular, the role of specialist mental health teams in supporting those with non-psychotic complex conditions is still disputed.

Case study: The Mental Health Link Project

The Mental Health Link project aimed to develop effective liaison between specialists and primary care and to develop shared care in response to the needs of patients, the practice, and the associated specialist mental health team (Byng and Single, 1999). The project also sought to establish processes for systematically reviewing patients in primary care. Facilitators met with a joint working group drawn from the CMHT and the practice in order to develop a shared care system from a selection of options contained in a toolkit. The two main focuses were firstly on the development of practice registers, minimum datasets for individual patients and recall systems and secondly, on the development of the link workers' role when they were away from their base community team working within general practice.

Evaluation of the Mental Health Link project involved a cluster randomised trial (Byng *et al*, 2004) and an evaluation involving qualitative interviews in order to understand the process of service development and the influence of the project (Byng *et al*, 2005).

Practice-CMHT vignettes have been composed from two or more of the original case studies. This approach facilitates the representation of the findings in narrative form without making the practices and associated CMHTs recognisable. The following vignettes, for example, focus on the various roles of link workers in caring for those with non-psychotic SEMI.

Vignette 1: integration of link worker achieved by helping solve crises and problems

A large practice with many GP partners in a relatively deprived inner-city area was allocated a link worker. The partners felt their case load warranted a practice-based CPN and, despite a strong interest in long-term mental illness (LTMI), they were suspicious that a link worker offering 2 hours a week would not contribute substantially. They found it difficult enough to meet as a team, and so meeting regularly as a group with the link worker was not an option.

However, in collaboration with the link worker, they worked out liaison arrangements to suit both sides. The link worker was introduced to the team in practice meetings and provided training to members of the PHCT on several occasions. He came into the practice weekly at a time when many of the team were in, and made himself available in the administrative hub of the practice as well as in quieter areas for in-depth consultations. He felt thoroughly welcomed by the practice and able to do a good and effective job. The practice on their part described him as a 'very special person', who would always take on their concerns and help solve a range of problems, including providing advice about complex patients with personality problems who were not in his trust's geographical area. He had experience of acute assessment as well as longer-term problems and knew the local services well. These attributes along with a willingness by the practice to collaborate resulted in effective reactive liaison in the absence of regular meetings.

Vignette 2: undue focus on continuing care stymies effective liaison

A small practice in an inner-city area recognised its need to improve care for patients with LTMI and decided to join the Mental Health Link programme. The GPs did not have particular interest or skills in primary care mental health, but wanted collaboration with CMHTs. The patients were evenly divided between CMHTs from two different trusts. Initially both CMHTs engaged with the project, but only one attended the first meeting. A link worker was appointed and it was agreed they would meet regularly with the practice.

Good relationships with the practice nurse and the GPs were maintained through informal contact with the continuing care team-based link worker. The joint meetings generated a trusting working relationship. There were a few patients with psychosis under the care of the continuing care team, but discussions about them became repetitive and after six months the meetings died out. The GPs, lacking confidence in dealing with difficult new mental health cases, realised in retrospect that they would have preferred to improve their links with the assessment and brief treatment team, so they could gain specialist input for those patients without psychosis but presenting with complex needs.

Vignette 3: liaison for proactive review

This medium-sized practice in an inner-city area, associated with a recently re-organised CMHT, had ambitions for developing practice-based shared care. However, when it came to planning the details of the liaison and the role of the link worker, the CMHT was reluctant to agree on a substantial role for the link worker other than as a channel for communication. In particular, the team voiced concerns that as the practice provided excellent mental healthcare, their priorities for liaison would lie elsewhere.

Meanwhile the practice itself underwent considerable disruption due to the loss of a partner. Over a year later the project was reviewed and a different link worker was appointed. The practice was more stable and, together, they worked out a system of joint review for all patients considered to have long-term mental illness. The practice manager organised one-to-one review meetings, with a list of patients, between the link worker and each of the GPs. Most of the patients discussed did not have psychosis. The reviews were rapid, with some patients who had been seen regularly and with few needs being discussed only briefly. The discussion of each patient ended with a decision about whether the patient:

- required no further immediate follow-up
- should be seen by the practice nurse for a physical health review
- should be seen by the GP for a mental health review
- should be referred to the CMHT.

Each patient's care was reviewed once or twice a year, and follow-up was targeted on those with most needs. The time allocated to these meetings was relatively limited, and the GPs respected the link worker as a limited resource by making initial contact with the care co-ordinators of patients under the trust in times of crisis, and reserving more complicated cases for discussion with the link worker.

Lessons from the vignettes

The vignettes show that a variety of approaches to liaison can improve care, but that liaison is not easy and there are many inhibiting factors. There is no one model that will fit all contexts. The needs of particular organisations, the context in which they are operating, and the needs of the patients all have to be taken into account when developing systems of shared care and liaison. Both sides need to be willing to engage, links are needed to support decisions which GPs were most unsure about, and the discussion of real cases led to the development of trusting relationships (Gilson, 2003). The consultation–liaison approach with all its theoretical advantages has not been widely adopted within the UK. The low number of psychiatrists per head of population means that it is impractical for each practice to have a linked psychiatrist. The case studies above, however, have shown that the 'consultation–liaison' approach can be carried out by experienced non-medical mental health specialist workers in a variety of ways.

Making it all happen

As has been suggested, there are currently few incentives in place to ensure that this important group of patients receives high standards of care within UK general practice.

The QOF component of the new GP contract now incorporates incentives to ensure that patients with new episodes of depression have their state assessed by a brief validated patient-centred assessment tool. There is, however, no incentive put in place to ensure an annual assessment for those with ongoing problems. This is likely to result in gaming, where people with recurrent depression and people with other problems who are depressed are classified as new-onset depressions (which technically they will be), so that there will be some incentive for people to have their mental state reviewed. It is possible that this will result in improvements in care along the lines outlined above. In the future it is hoped that the QOF will incorporate incentives for reviewing those with long-term, non-psychotic mental health conditions.

The importance of this group must come to the attention of commissioners before the problem is fully addressed. Practice-based commissioning and payment-by-results may result in significant service redesign. As care is brought closer to patients' homes, and specialists are brought into primary care mental health teams, it will be easier to ensure that specialist input is focused more on those with chronic mental health problems of a non-psychotic nature as well as those with psychosis.

A further government-led priority is to get people back into work. It is now recognised that there are significant hurdles for people with mental health problems to overcome before they become more involved in the workforce, but that with additional support it is possible to encourage people back to work. The interventions designed primarily to bring people back into the workforce may have spin-offs in terms of improving the overall care of people with chronic, non-psychotic conditions.

Conclusion

In conclusion, severe and enduring mental illness extends to illnesses such as longstanding depression, anxiety and a variety of other conditions that currently have high levels of symptoms and disability, and care provision is systematically poor in terms of review and opportunities for psychosocial interventions. In this chapter, I have outlined ways in which practitioners can work with individuals over time, and have suggested changes to systems that will enable this to occur more efficiently. There are significant opportunities in the future, which may help to ensure that these changes occur.

References

Andrews G (2001) Should depression be managed as a chronic disease? *British Medical Journal* 322:419–21.

Andrews G, Sanderson K and Beard J (1998) Burden of disease. Methods of calculating disability from mental disorder. *British Journal of Psychiatry* 173:123–31.

Arnow BA and Constantino MJ (2003) Effectiveness of psychotherapy and combination treatment for chronic depression. *Journal of Clinical Psychology* 59:893–905.

Bindman J, Johnson S, Wright S *et al* (1997) Integration between primary and secondary services in the care of the severely mentally ill: patients' and general practitioners' views. *British Journal of Psychiatry* 171:169–74.

Byng R, Jones R, Leese M *et al* (2004) Exploratory cluster randomised controlled trial of shared care development for long-term mental illness. *British Journal of General Practice* 54:259–66.

Byng R, Norman I and Redfern S (2005) Using realistic evaluation to evaluate a practice level intervention to improve primary health care for patients with long-term mental illness. *Evaluation* 11:69–93.

Byng R and Single H (1999) *Developing Primary Care for Patients with Long Term Mental Illness – your guide to improving services.* London: King's Fund.

Catalan J, Gath D, Bond A *et al* (1988) General practice patients on long-term psychotropic drugs. A controlled investigation. *British Journal of Psychiatry* 152:399–405.

Clinical Governance Resource Group (2004) *Lewisham Mental Health Facilitation Project Progress Report.* London: South-east London Clinical Governance Resource Group.

Copeland ME (2005) *Wellness Recovery Action Plan: a system for monitoring, reducing and eliminating uncomfortable or dangerous physical symptoms.* Liverpool: Sefton Recovery Group.

Craft LL and Landers DM (1998) The effect of exercise on clinical depression and depression resulting from mental illness. A meta-analysis. *Journal of Sport and Exercise Psychology* 20:339–57.

Creed F and Marks B (1989) Liaison psychiatry in general practice: a comparison of the liaison-attachment scheme and shifted outpatient clinic models. *Journal of the Royal College of General Practitioners* 39:514–17.

Department of Health (1994) *Working in Partnership: The review of mental health nursing.* London: HMSO.

Freeth R (2004) *Psychopharmacology, and Counselling and Psychotherapy.* Information Sheet for the British Association for Counselling and Psychotherapy (BACP). Rugby: British Association for Counselling and Psychotherapy.

Gask L, Sibbald B and Creed F (1997) Evaluating models of working at the interface between mental health services and primary care. *British Journal of Psychiatry* 170:6–11.

Gilson L (2003) Trust and the development of health care as a social institution. *Social Science and Medicine* 56:1453–68.

Goldberg D and Gournay K (1997) *The General Practitioner, the Psychiatrist and the Burden of Mental Health Care.* (No.1) Maudsley Discussion Paper. London: Institute of Psychiatry.

Harrison J, Kisely SR, Jones JA, Blake I and Creed FH (1997) Access to psychiatric care; the results of the pathways to care study in Preston. *Journal of Public Health Medicine* 19:69–75.

Joint Royal College Working Group (1993) *Shared Care of Patients with Mental Health Problems.* Occasional Paper 60. London: Royal College of General Practitioners.

Kai J, Crosland A and Drinkwater C (2000) Prevalence of enduring and disabling mental illness in the inner city. *British Journal of General Practice* 50:992–4.

Kendrick T, Burns T, Freeling P and Sibbald B (1994) Provision of care to general practice patients with disabling long-term mental illness: a survey in 16 practices. *British Journal of General Practice* 44:301–5.

Lauber C, Nordt C, Falcato L and Rossler W (2001) Lay recommendations on how to treat mental disorders. *Social Psychiatry and Psychiatric Epidemiology* 36:553–6.

Launer J (2002) *Narrative-based Primary Care. A practical guide.* Oxford: Radcliffe Medical Press.

Mitchell AR (1985) Psychiatrists in primary health care settings. *British Journal of Psychiatry* 147:371–9.

Office for National Statistics (2005) *Labour Force Survey.* London: Office for National Statistics.

Patients as Teachers Research Team (2003) *Shared decision-making? Patients' views about their treatment for depression in Primary Care. A qualitative research study.* Lewisham: Lewisham Primary Care Trust.

Pullen IM and Yellowlees AJ (1988) Scottish psychiatrists in primary health-care settings. A silent majority. *British Journal of Psychiatry* 153:663–6.

Ritchie JH, Dick D and Lingham R (1994) *Report of the Enquiry into the Care and Treatment of Christopher Clunis.* London: HMSO.

Rogers A and Pilgrim D (2003) *Mental Health and Inequality.* Basingstoke: Palgrave Macmillan.

Sayce L, Craig TKJ and Boardman AP (1991) The development of community mental health centres in the UK. *Social Psychiatry and Psychiatric Epidemiology* 26:14–20.

Schwenk TL, Evans DL, Laden SK and Lewis L (2004) Treatment outcome and physician–patient communication in primary care patients with chronic, recurrent depression. *American Journal of Psychiatry* 161:1892–901.

Slade M, Powell R and Strathdee G (1997) Current approaches to identifying the severely mentally ill. *Social Psychiatry and Psychiatric Epidemiology* 32:177–84.

Strathdee G (1988) Psychiatrists in primary care: the general practitioner viewpoint. *Family Practice* 5:111–15.

Strathdee G and Williams P (1984) A survey of psychiatrists in primary care: the silent growth of a new service. *Journal of the Royal College of General Practitioners* 34:615–18.

Thomas RVR and Corney RH (1992) A survey of links between mental health professionals and general practice in six district health authorities. *British Journal of General Practice* 42:358–61.

Von Korff M and Goldberg D (2001) Improving outcomes in depression. *British Medical Journal* 323:948–9.

Vuorilehto M, Melartin T and Isometsa E (2005) Depressive disorders in primary care: recurrent, chronic, and co-morbid. *Psychological Medicine* 35:673–82.

Wagner EH (1998) Chronic disease management: what will it take to improve care for chronic illness? *Effective Clinical Practice* 1:2–4.

Wagner EH, Austin BT and Von Korff M (1996) Improving outcomes in chronic illness. *Managed Care Quarterly* 4:12–25.

Williams P and Balestrieri M (1989) Psychiatric clinics in general practice. Do they reduce admissions? *British Journal of Psychiatry* 154:67–71.

Chapter 6

Severe and enduring mental illness in relation to discrimination, racism, prejudice, ethnicity and culture

Maurice Lipsedge

Introduction

This chapter deals with the delivery of healthcare to people with chronic, enduring mental illness in relation to discrimination, racism, prejudice, ethnicity and culture. Each of these terms can be defined in various ways (Mason, 2000). I will use the following working definitions:

Discrimination is behaviour that systematically disfavours or treats harshly members of one particular group who are more or less conspicuously different. Discrimination is the practical expression of *prejudice*, which can itself be defined as a knee-jerk, negative perception of a person triggered by one or more aspects of a person's ethnicity such as their religious affiliation.

Racism is a particular type of discrimination that is based on inherited physical attributes most commonly skin colour.

Ethnicity is a complex notion as it is made up of a variety of factors that can include one or more of the following:

- religion
- inherited physical characteristics
- place of birth
- language
- dialect
- culture (*see* below).

The term '*ethnic minority*' might refer to a group of people on the basis of their skin colour, their religion, their language or their shared history, or any combination of these. The word 'ethnic' is derived from the Greek *ethnikos*, which actually means a heathen, and in Middle English this word came to denote a person who adhered to neither the Christian nor the Jewish faith (Pearsall, 1998).

By the same token the term *Kaffir*, which is actually an offensive word used in South Africa to denote a black African, is derived from the Arabic word *kafir*, which among Muslims refers to a person who is not a Muslim, i.e. an infidel or an unbeliever.

So, historically, the term ethnic was itself used ethnocentrically, i.e. to evaluate other cultures according to preconceptions originating in one's own culture.

It is obvious that each of these terms can be difficult to define with any degree of precision. How does a person who left their country of birth in childhood, who is bilingual and whose parents belong to a different religion define their own ethnic identity? Ethnic classification by oneself or by others will vary according to the salience given to one or more of these diverse criteria. Medical and psychological publications routinely use demographic terms that conflate and conceal (Hicks, 2004). For example, in the US, the term 'Asian' usually refers to people of Chinese, Japanese or South East Asian origin. In this country, the same term might be used to cover people as diverse as a man whose grandparents were born in Tamil Nadu and whose parents were born in Singapore, or a woman born in East London whose parents have migrated from Sylhet in Bangladesh. Classification by religious affiliation is equally problematic because it fails to recognise the spectrum from orthodoxy to secularism and divisions within religious denominations, e.g. Seventh Day Adventists, Baptists and Greek Orthodox are all Christians. Classification by place of birth, i.e. by geography does not help either. What does it mean nowadays to be Sudanese or to be Iraqi or to be American?

The definition of *culture* is even more contentious. A useful construct is to regard culture as a bundle of attitudes, expectations, beliefs and practices that an individual acquires during their socialisation, initially within their family and later during their education and their contact with society at large. Some people will, of course, reject their culture of origin and/or embrace a new one, or create some sort of amalgamation or syncretism, and sometimes psychiatrists conflate race and culture. For example, in his introduction to descriptive psychopathology, Andrew Sims correctly emphasises the importance of culture in evaluating the significance of a possible schizophrenic delusion of control, but inadvertently refers to the need to take account of the patient's 'racial background' (Sims, 1988).

According to the biopsychosocial model which now dominates the practice of psychiatry, the salience of neurophysiological understanding has to be tempered with knowledge and understanding gained from both the psychological and social sciences. Within the psychosocial framework, the past two decades have witnessed increasing attention to cultural factors (Littlewood and Lipsedge, 1997).

An awareness of cultural diversity has to inform the assessment of psychopathology. In particular one has to be aware of the fact that idioms of distress might be culturally specific (Kleinman and Good, 1985). To what extent do the current standardised diagnostic systems (ICD-10 (World Health Organization, 1992) and DSM IV (American Psychiatric Association, 1994)), which have been developed in a Western industrialised setting, have validity in non-Western cultures? A mental health worker who relies exclusively on the use of Western culture-specific diagnostic categories might either pathologise culturally important patterns of distress, or dismiss them as irrelevant 'noise' or otherwise deride them. (The word noise in communication technology refers to 'irregular fluctuations accompanying and tending to *obscure* [emphasis added] electrical signals or other significant phenomena' (*Concise Oxford Dictionary*, 2002).)

Each culture has its own culturally prescribed lexicon for expressing illness and misfortune, including severe chronic psychiatric disorder, and for defining the optimal treatment for that particular person in that specific situation (Kleinman, 1988).

The idiom of the explanations of the likely cause of mental health problems might be:

- supernatural, e.g. spirit intrusion, soul loss
- religious
- moralistic, e.g. punishment for sin, breach of taboo, neglect of ancestors, etc
- naturalistic, e.g. humoral imbalance (Helman, 2001).

Although it is known that people living in traditional cultures might have different ways of labelling discomfort, disability, pain and distress, and of seeking help to alleviate these conditions, the continuing influence of traditional beliefs after migration into contemporary Western society and into subsequent generations has not yet been clearly delineated (*see* Bhugra *et al*, 1999).

Culture determines the interpretation by the individual and his or her family of pain, discomfort or distress as to whether it merits the application of a household folk remedy or a consultation with a practitioner or healer, or indeed whether it merits any attention at all. In summary, culture determines the transformation from a person to a patient and will influence the decision as to whether to seek help from a medical or a non-medical source (Kleinman, 1980).

In-depth interviews or 'illness narratives', an approach not unfamiliar to counsellors and psychotherapists, provide information not only about the individual's subjective and interpersonal world but also about the patient's and their family's Explanatory Model (Kleinman, 1988). An example of a cross-cultural, in-depth narrative interview is the encounter with Nepali-speaking refugees from Bhutan who employed metaphors to express distress (Sharma and Van Ommeren, 1998). These interviews also revealed how the Hindu torture survivors used *karma* as an explanation for suffering, and how this interpretation could contribute to positive coping.

Cultural and demographic factors which affect the therapeutic encounter include not only the obvious distance between interviewer and client that might arise from differences in sex, ethnicity, socio-economic status, urban/rural background and citizenship status, but also whether deference and acquiescence are socially desirable or whether the interview itself is perceived as intrusive or stigmatising. Other cultural factors that can affect the interview include the optimal interpersonal distance, the norms of privacy and whether questions have to be asked in both the positive and negative form (de Jong and Van Ommeren, 2002).

The cross-cultural interview might fail to reveal important information for the following reasons:

- fear on the part of the therapist of being intrusive and causing offence means that significant questions may be avoided on sensitive topics like:
  - personal and sexual relationships
  - adherence to strict religious beliefs and practices
  - independence from the extended family
  - conflict between the generations
  - the public expression of piety and conformity
- lack of awareness about cultural practices might lead to the false assumption that a situation of actual abuse is merely a feature of the culture, as in the mistreatment of Victoria Climbié, where vital matters were falsely attributed to cultural norms and remained unexplored (Laming, 2003)

- cross-cultural matching of therapist and client cannot guarantee full disclosure about an abusive situation such as domestic violence. An abused client might be too ashamed and embarrassed to report abuse to a practitioner from a similar background. Conversely, although a sense of group loyalty might inhibit disclosure to an outsider, the latter's 'otherness' might actually facilitate this (Kareem and Littlewood, 2000)
- 'category fallacy'. This is an influential concept introduced into cross-cultural psychiatry by Arthur Kleinman (1987), an anthropologist/psychiatrist, to draw attention to the situation where a psychological construct is not translatable into another language because it lacks cross-cultural meaning or relevance.

The ethnographic research by Alison Spiro, a health visitor working with Gujarati, Hindu and Jain families in Harrow, North West London, reveals the role of supernatural beliefs in lay models of the causation of illness. Beliefs in the evil eye (*najar*) and ghosts (*bhut*) and the practice of specific rituals to protect the vulnerable have been transmitted through generations and across three continents, i.e. from India, via East Africa to the UK. People are thought to be most at risk of attack by the evil eye during transitional phases of the life cycle, i.e. marriage, pregnancy, childbirth and childhood, so it is at these periods of heightened vulnerability that *najar* has to be detected and thwarted (Spiro, 2005).

In order to establish a culture-informed approach, we need culture-specific qualitative data or 'thick' descriptions to help us to understand the socio-cultural context. In a provocative paper on 'lying', the Canadian anthropologist Massé describes how health-seeking behaviour can be determined by a cultural context which might include a belief in the efficacy of supernatural mediation. In his study of local folk healers in the Caribbean, the *gadés* and *quimboiseurs* of Martinique and St Lucia, Massé describes the encounter between the ill person and the traditional healer 'as a meeting of two discourses that more or less consciously integrate truths and lies, frankness (*franchise*) and deception for the production of a dynamic truth' (Massé, 2002, p. 176). In these French Creole societies disease, mental illness and personal problems are attributed to supernatural forces unleashed by an evil spell cast by a *gadé* or *quimboiseur* at the request of a jealous or envious person. The victim of this witchcraft consults the *gadé* or *quimboiseur*, who takes on the reverse role of traditional healer. The healer then mobilises supernatural forces to undo the evil spell. The *gadé's* credibility has been acquired through a natural gift, a revelation or an apprenticeship. Misfortune, bad behaviour and depressive hallucinations are attributed by the victims to the malign work of hostile spirits, and the traditional healers confirm that their clients are not responsible for their acts, 'their minds being altered by the work of an evil spirit sent by a jealous person' (Massé, 2002, p. 177). The client disowns responsibility for their behaviour and their misfortunes while the highly paid healer arrogates and articulates a supernatural power (Massé, 2002, p. 177).

Massé points out that in the contemporary francophone Caribbean pluralist medical context, people have access to a wide variety of healthcare systems including professional help from biomedical physicians, Pentecostal pastors and charismatic priests. However, there is a bias in favour of traditional healing practices and supernatural explanations for misfortune. These magico-religious beliefs are part of a cultural heritage that suddenly and uncontrollably rises to the surface in times of crisis (Massé, 2002, p. 186). In choosing a *gadé/quimboiseur* from a range of potential healing agents, the patient selects a system which absolves him or her of personal guilt by identifying external causes (i.e. witchcraft) motivated by envy or spite. Massé asks provocatively whether the sick person is 'lying' when they blame evil spirits for their unacceptable behaviour, and whether the healer is merely taking advantage of his client's credulity (Massé, 2002, p. 175). Massé suggests that pastors, *quimboiseurs* and biomedical physicians all adjust their discourse to fit into the patient's beliefs (Massé, 2002, p. 178).

Racism and mental health

The psychological impact of racist experiences has been comprehensively reviewed by Bhugra and Ayonrinde (2001) and Bhugra and Cochrane (2001), who delineate a pathway from the experience of racism to the development of common mental disorders, especially of depression. These authors draw on both sociological and psychological research that has established the role of major adverse life events and of the systematic undermining of self-esteem in the aetiology of depression. Victimisation by prejudice and discrimination induces a sense of entrapment and humiliation, which can lead to the helpless despair and profound pessimism that characterise some depressive illnesses. Immigrants, whether involuntary, as in the case of refugees, or elective, economically motivated migrants, might be sustained by the prospect of safety or of a higher standard of living, but their security or their job prospects will be undermined by selectively harsh treatment from members of the host community or by other ethnic groups (Bhughra and Jones, 2001). A sense of pervasive vulnerability is engendered by discrimination based on an immutable visible physical feature such as skin colour. The 'black' or 'brown' person in a predominantly 'white' area experiences two contrasting problems with anonymity. Their individual identity might be denied by other people because of their obvious membership of a different ethnic group. Conversely, they themselves are denied the safety of anonymity in a crowd. An urban ecological study of psychosis in immigrants has shown that having neighbours from the same background acts as a protective factor (Boydell *et al*, 2001).

Factors that contribute to the causative pathway from racism to overt mental health problems include enhanced vulnerability associated with low self-esteem, major adverse life events such as a racially motivated assault or an unjustified stop-and-search, in addition to long-term difficulties that members of ethnic minorities might share with their 'white' neighbours in terms of poor housing, unemployment or unsatisfactory jobs. The possible protective role of a system-blaming perspective and of a strong ethnic identity has not yet been clearly established by social and psychological research.

The cumulative experience of racially motivated mistreatment can affect physical as well as mental health. A 13-year study of the health of African-Americans showed an excess of cardiovascular disease which was particularly pronounced in those who had endured a disproportionate amount of racist mistreatment (Jackson *et al*, 1996).

Most mental health professionals would claim to be free of racist attitudes and behaviour. But racist assumptions may be subtle and might be unrecognised by psychiatrists, nurses and psychotherapists. It is obvious that the attitudes and utterances of people at a psychiatric facility, whether it is a community mental health centre, an open ward, an intensive care unit, a medium secure or a secure unit, will invariably reflect the perceptions and verbal practices of the outside world and of the broader community.

I remember visiting prisoners on remand on the medical wing at Wandsworth Prison in the 1970s and noticing that some of the prison officers were wearing National Front tie pins. With the amendment to the Race Relations Act, blatant racist intimidation of that type is challenged although there is obviously a great deal more to be done. Although it might be argued that the expression of prejudice and acts of discrimination have become less overt over the past generation, it would be absurd to claim that the problem has been eradicated.

Why is verbal racist abuse so damaging? After all, our parents will have tried to reassure all of us with the old-fashioned saying: 'Sticks and stones will break my bones but names will never hurt me'. But names do hurt and they hurt profoundly. We know from studies of the impact of bullying that the most psychologically damaging form of verbal harassment consists of insults about any conspicuous physical feature of the victim (Leyman, 1996). So, it follows that verbal abuse that refers to an immutable characteristic of the victim's anatomy or histology is highly destructive and a threat to that person's self-esteem. Since one of the main therapeutic aims of psychiatry should be the restoration or the enhancement of a patient's self-esteem, a psychiatric ward environment in which racist abuse is condoned or tolerated or disregarded, is demonstrably counter-therapeutic. None of us can change our skin colour and if that colour is publicly and repeatedly devalued, the victim will feel both powerless and helpless. Together with damaged self-esteem, psychiatric patients already have to cope with a sense of powerlessness and entrapment. Schizophrenia can make the sufferer feel that they are the passive victim of threatening, menacing or derogatory voices and that they are the target of persecution and of secret conspiracies. It is self-evident that racist abuse will compound this feeling of persecution. It will also enhance the sense of powerlessness, because there is nothing that we can do to change those anatomical features that are devalued by racism and by racists. The first incident in the sequence of events that led to the death during restraint of David Bennett (*see Independent Inquiry into the Death of David Bennett*, 2003) at a medium secure unit was the fact that he was called a 'black bastard'. The conjunction of the word 'black' with 'bastard' is important. The term 'bastard' has, in addition to the original meaning of illegitimate, the following connotations: misbegotten, inferior, substandard, low grade, second rate, subnormal, imperfect, inadequate, deficient.

If there is a climate in a mental health facility where profoundly damaging expressions such as this are tolerated or are disregarded by medical or nursing staff, or are given low priority by the managers, then the clients will take their cue in the sense that those patients with racist attitudes will feel that it is OK to express them, while the targets of racist comments will feel unsupported and devalued. In fact they will feel dehumanised or 'objectified'. *Objectification* is the term coined by Frantz Fanon, the French West Indian psychiatrist, who, of course, experienced racism himself and who described his Algerian patients' experience of prejudice and discrimination. In answer to the question: 'What does racism do to people?' Fanon replied that racism confines, it imprisons, it hardens and it objectifies, i.e. it makes a person into a thing and a thing by definition has no capacity for human relationships (Schmitt, 1996). Fanon describes how racism achieves this objectification (*'choseification'*) by the processes of infantilisation, denigration, distrust, ridicule, exclusion, scapegoating and rendering invisible. Fanon did not want the unique complexity of a person to be summed up by and reduced to the colour of their skin.

A failure to acknowledge more subtle aspects of racism and racist assumptions can undermine psychotherapeutic activity (Bhugra and Bhui, 1998). In *Intercultural Therapy* by the late Jafar Kareem and Roland Littlewood (2000), Lennox Thomas gives the following vignette: a young black woman on her way to her psychotherapy session was spat on and called names like 'nigger' by an elderly white woman in a bus queue. She arrived at her white female psychotherapist's consulting room in a tearful and distressed state. On telling the psychotherapist that she had called the woman 'a wicked old cow' the psychotherapist's first response was that she should not have reacted in this way because the woman was elderly. The psychotherapist's view was that the best way of dealing with this incident would have been for the black patient to ignore it. The patient responded by feeling angry but she was unable to express this anger until several sessions later. She felt that her psychotherapist was not concerned about her feelings and that she was being protective to another white person whom the psychotherapist did not even know. She now perceived that her psychotherapist, who had been treating her for many months, still did not have any real concern for her or any real comprehension of her situation. She abruptly terminated therapy because she felt that the psychotherapist had no true understanding of her patient's feelings and that she had merely demonstrated an instinctive solidarity with another, in this case unknown, white person rather than make any effort to grasp the meaning of this young woman's distress which had been caused by an explicit racist verbal assault (Thomas, 2000).

For at least the past decade, the Mental Health Act Commission has produced a training pack on race and culture. This draws attention to the fact that both black patients and black staff are often unwilling to complain openly about racism to commissioners because they feel that their complaints may not be taken seriously. The report on the death of Orville Blackwood at Broadmoor refers to patients' reluctance to discuss racism for fear of being dismissed as deluded (Special Hospital Service Authority, 1993; Lipsedge, 1994). In their policy document on race and culture published round about the same time, the Mental Health Act Commission advised their visiting team members to check whether medical and nursing staff were aware of the possible effects of ethnic stereotyping on estimates of dangerousness.

Stigma and somatisation

Hussain and Cochrane (2004) have critically reviewed a number of claims about cultural and religious factors that might affect the recognition of mental illness in South Asians, i.e. Bangladeshi, Indian and Pakistani and Sri Lankan people living in this country. These often unquestioned claims frequently refer to three major themes: stigma, somatisation and the use of traditional healers and religion as treatment for depression.

There has been a widespread assumption among GPs and other clinicians that

Asian patients tend to express their psychological problems in physical terms. In fact, there is little difference in the rates of somatising between Asian and indigenous patients (Goldberg *et al*, 1988).

A common reason adduced for the under-utilisation of mental health services by individuals from South Asia is the greater stigma that they attach to mental illness (Nazroo, 1997). In fact, such stigma is universal and it reduces the marriage prospects for people from all communities. The question of the relative duration of delay in seeking help for mental illness in families remains to be resolved. A study of Chinese caregivers in Toronto showed that they were more likely to keep mental illness in the family a secret from others. They were more reluctant to seek psychiatric treatment for a relative with mental illness than 'Euro-Canadians', resulting in a relatively longer interval between the onset of symptoms and initiation of treatment (Ryder *et al*, 2000). This led to a greater perceived burden, i.e. the Chinese families took longer to seek treatment after the onset of prominent psychotic symptoms. They also reported a higher number of burdensome behaviours, e.g. self-neglect, reclusiveness and the need for close supervision.

It has been suggested that within Chinese culture, mental illness stigmatises the entire family so that it is concealed and contained within the family for as long as possible. In addition to stigma, another cause of delay in seeking help might be the perception that mental illness, with its severely disruptive effects on family life, requires a family approach rather than outside intervention. This makes sense in terms of the traditional Chinese emphasis on the parent–child bond, and on the central role of the family as the focal point for socialisation and collective responsibility (Ryder *et al*, 2000).

A culturally sensitive approach to mental health problems

The use of cultural formulations in psychiatric diagnosis helps the practitioner to negotiate across the gulf between their own world view, which might be a secular one, and the patient's universe, which might be dominated by supernatural constructs which are not shared by the practitioner (*see* Heilman and Witztum, 2000).

A detailed example is the case history of Mr A, a 57-year-old Chinese American engineer whose first contact with a psychiatrist occurred after he had experienced auditory hallucinations and delusions for a period of three weeks. These unusual experiences, which were labelled as schizophreniform, had started shortly after Mr A had begun to extensively practise *Qi-Gong* for recurrent back pain. *Qi-Gong* is a Chinese folk health-enhancing practice which requires controlled synchronised breathing and body movements. Mr A began to hear the voices of a supernatural being instructing him on how to practise *Qi-Gong*, and he started to believe that he was able to contact entities from another dimension (Lim and Lin, 1996).

He was treated with a low dose of haloperidol (an antipsychotic drug), and simultaneously he stopped the practice of *Qi-Gong* because he felt that it was not helping him. Mr A's auditory hallucinations and delusional beliefs persisted although they lost some of their distressing quality. Nevertheless, his symptoms were sufficiently distracting to prevent Mr A from returning to work. After two months Mr A insisted on stopping the medication.

The cultural formulation takes into account the patient's cultural identity, cultural explanations of his illness, cultural factors related to his psychosocial environment and cultural elements of the clinician–patient relationship. Mr A identified strongly with both his Chinese heritage and his adopted country in the US. He was regarded by his Chinese American psychiatrist as 'fully bicultural', having adapted to mainstream American society while maintaining ties with the Chinese American community. He was fluent in both the Fukien dialect and Mandarin, as well as English which was the language of the clinical encounter with a Chinese-Canadian therapist, although he used Mandarin when he found that English could not adequately convey some of the meaning of his experiences (Lim and Lin, 1996).

Mr A was born in Fukien province and moved with his parents and family to Taiwan in 1949. As a young man he migrated to the US, where he obtained a postgraduate degree. He got married in the US. He watches both American and Chinese language television and reads both English and Chinese language newspapers. He is familiar with folk-healing methods but in general prefers Western medicine. He spends time at work and socially with both Chinese-American and American-born people of other ethnicities.

The cultural explanations of his illness considered Mr A's symptoms in relation to his Chinese health model, notably the corporeal circulation of the vital force of *Qi* through special channels (Lim and Lin, 1996).

Medical pluralism

In traditional non-Western societies there are both medical and non-medical frameworks for dealing with mental health problems (Kleinman, 1980).

People with personal problems or with psychiatric disorders, and their carers, can hold mutually contradictory beliefs about the cause and appropriate actions to be taken to deal with their affliction. Thus, naturalistic models such as viral infections or vitamin deficiency can co-exist with personalistic explanations as exemplified by supernatural influences, sin and punishment, and *karma*. A patient from Africa or Asia or South America might both consult a traditional healer and take antipsychotic medication, just as an English patient might supplement their standard medication with homoeopathic and herbal drugs now widely sold in one large chain of retail stores as 'Boots Alternatives'.

Tanya Crawford has described how psychological distress is identified and explained among Zulu people and how traditional healers understand their role and treatment methods. Zulu people consult traditional healers (diviners, faith healers or herbalists) as well as Western doctors to treat mental illness and distress. While Western biomedicine is seen as useful in providing treatment, diviners and faith healers are particularly valued for their skills in identifying the cause of illness, and patients and their families tend to shop around for a practitioner who gives advice that is in keeping with their own beliefs. Psychological distress is usually explained in terms of sorcery, displeasure from the ancestors or social causes. Traditional Zulu healers use treatment aimed at harmonising the patient with their environment through neutralising sorcery, appeasing ancestors or directly manipulating the environment (Crawford and Lipsedge, 2004).

Insight

Psychiatrists, mainly of British white ethnic origin, are more inclined to attribute insight to patients from their own backgrounds than to patients of a different ethnicity. In a study of 357 patients with a psychotic illness admitted to an inner-London psychiatric hospital, it was found that black African and black Caribbean patients were judged by doctors to have significantly less insight than British white patients (Johnson and Orrell, 1996, pp. 1081–4). A number of explanations have been offered for this perceived association between insight and ethnicity. First, there are different ways of understanding mental distress, abnormal experience and mental illness in different cultures, i.e. there may be a culture-bound perception of the nature and presentation of mental illness which is different from the Western biomedical model. These differences can have a marked influence on the mental health worker's attitude or the doctor's diagnostic practice.

Secondly and controversially, in some cultures there might be a greater stigma attached to mental illness, and a greater fear of the treatment provided by psychiatrists. This in turn can lead to denial of the illness and a reluctance to have early contact with the mental health services. As a result, by the time of admission, the condition of patients such as these has deteriorated to the extent that insight is more likely to be lost.

There may also be linguistic barriers to the accurate assessment of insight. Furthermore, the psychiatrist's rating of insight might be affected by their own perceptions and expectations of patients from certain ethnic groups, who are assumed to lack awareness of their own mental illness (Johnson and Orrell, 1996).

Saravanan *et al* (2004) have developed a model of insight that tries to avoid 'eurocentricity' by taking cultural idioms into account and by recognising 'medical pluralism'. They propose a cross-culturally valid working model of insight: '. . . if a person could acknowledge some kind of non-visible change in his or her body or mind that affects the ability to function socially, and if he or she feels the need for restitution, then irrespective of the attribution and the pathways of care that a person seeks, we could call this the presence of "insight"' (Saravanan *et al*, 2004, p. 108).

Religion

As Kate Loewenthal (1995) has succinctly written in her invaluable handbook *Religion and Mental Health*: '. . . clients may perceive psychotherapy and psychotherapists as a totally Godless crew' (p. 156). Psychotherapists might be regarded as both insensitive and ignorant of their clients' religious beliefs, values and practices. They might also be perceived as frankly negative or even hostile about these matters. Secular psychotherapists and counsellors might be averse to religion, and dismissive of the positive and adaptive role of spirituality in the way people deal with existential matters, i.e. life, death and meaning. Furthermore, clients may fear that their beliefs and practices might be regarded as suggestive of psychopathology.

American psychiatrists and psychologists and other mental health professionals are more inclined to label themselves as agnostic, atheist or humanist than the population at large (Coyle, 2001), and this generalisation probably applies to British mental health workers. More psychiatrists give up religious beliefs than adopt them, and psychiatry itself has aspired to an empirical basis which has, by definition, completely excluded the supernatural. This, of course, is at odds with the world view of many of their patients.

An awareness of how distress can be articulated through the medium of religion is shown in an incisive paper entitled 'All in faith: religion as the idiom and means of coping with distress', by Heilman and Witztum (2000). This demonstrates how the practitioner's knowledge of the central role of religious beliefs and practices in their patients' lives can narrow the gulf between the secular ideology of psychiatry and the religious fundamentalism of their patients. Acquiring relevant ethnographic knowledge is essential for establishing a therapeutic alliance with a patient from an unfamiliar background.

As an example of the need to be circumspect when making a mental health assessment of an adherent to an unfamiliar and numerically small religious sect, consider the Jewish ultra-orthodox messianic sect described by Simon Dein (2002, 2004). The Lubavitch Hasidim of Stamford Hill, North London, constitute one subdivision of the broader spectrum of fundamentalist orthodox Jews. They revere their semi-hereditary spiritual leader whose blessing and advice are sought to deal with transitional crises such as a decision to marry, failure to conceive or the diagnosis of a grave illness. Consulting the Rebbe in this way is a time-honoured procedure and is regarded as 'mainstream' within this statistically small congregation. Dein describes from first-hand ethnographic observation the recent emergence of a collective belief that the terminally ill Rabbi Schneerson was in fact the Messiah. This belief, which is heterodox and shocking to the point of anathema for most orthodox Jews, has animated hundreds of the Rebbe's followers. Some of his devotees have waited in hopeful anticipation of Rabbi Schneerson's emergence as the Messiah by denying the fact of his death. However, the majority of the sect have rationalised his death and the subsequent failure of the Millennium to materialise as evidence of their own unworthiness. In terms of the standard psychiatric textbook's definition of a delusion, those who deny that Rabbi Schneerson is dead meet the first three criteria for a delusional belief, i.e.:

1 an unshakeable belief
2 held with great conviction
3 despite evidence to the contrary – in this case the well-publicised death of the Rebbe and his non-resurrection.

What about the fourth criterion for a delusion, i.e. that it is a belief that is not shared by other members of the person's social, cultural and religious background? In the case of the Stamford Hill Lubavitch congregation, a vocal but numerically small subgroup do indeed share this belief, so a mental health worker would conventionally have to fall back on group membership as a way of avoiding unnecessary (and harmful) 'pathologisation'. By convention, any 'successful' religious innovator, with success being measured by the evolution of a viable band of followers, might be spared a psychiatric label (but *see* Littlewood 1983, 1984).

Thus, Jonathan Martin, the lone pious Christian Evangelical fundamentalist who tried to burn down York Minster in 1829 in response to prophetic dreams, was a loner who was and is regarded as insane (Lipsedge, 2003) whereas his near-contemporary, Joanna Southcott, who claimed that she was pregnant with the Second Coming, attracted a band of followers, perhaps because she did nothing antisocial (Harrison, 1979).

Schizophrenia and culture

When assessing the symptoms of schizophrenia in patients from unfamiliar cultures, clinicians must take into account culture-specific factors that might lead to misdiagnosis. Thus, a psychiatrist from overseas who elicited from an elderly English patient the fact that to cure her infertility she had gone to Dorset to sit on a giant's penis concluded that she was deluded. He was unaware of the magic potency of the Rude Giant of Cerne Abbas.

Research has shown that lower socio-economic status, African-American and Hispanic patients are disproportionately more likely to be given a diagnosis of schizophrenia when a diagnosis of bipolar affective disorder might be more appropriate. Cultural factors might influence most aspects of schizophrenia (*see* Jenkins, 1998) including the identification, personal and social meaning of this psychotic illness as well as the form, content and constellation of schizophrenic symptoms. It has also been established that the course, social outcome and utilisation of treatment for this condition can be affected by the individual's culture (Jenkins, 1998). Both the clinician's and the patient's cultural baggage and presuppositions will influence their appraisal of each other and of their respective appearance, behaviour, speech and affect.

Jenkins, who is both a psychiatrist and an anthropologist, refers to the observation that in schizophrenia there is often a disruption in the person's sense of self as a circumscribed and boundaried individual who is autonomous and self-directed. However, this sense of self is a Euro-American culture-specific construct, and she emphasises the importance of assessing any expression of a breach of this 'envelope' in terms of the individual's cultural context (Jenkins, 1998; *see* also Jenkins and Barrett, 2004).

Jenkins also helpfully draws attention to the frequency of 'normal-range' visual hallucinatory experiences which are a regular part of everyday experience in Latin American cultures. In general, visual and auditory hallucinations, e.g. hearing God's voice, might be 'culturally normative' in some Asian, African and Latin American contexts (Jenkins, 1998). Some cultures may actually value rather than pathologise hallucinatory experiences when they occur in a socially sanctioned context (Littlewood and Lipsedge, 1997).

Culture might affect both the structure and content of schizophrenic disorders. In schizophrenia there is often flattening of affect which is characterised by facial immobility and lack of responsiveness with poor eye contact and reduced expressive body language. However, as Jenkins (1998) points out, cultures vary in their typical mode of emotional expressions which might also be significantly different when the clinical interviewer is not of the same sex as the patient or client. Both culture and sex might influence the style of display of affect (Jenkins, 1998).

Furthermore, some widely held, culturally sanctioned beliefs might be regarded as delusional in another cultural context, e.g. the Roman Catholic doctrine of trans-substantiation according to which the substance of the Eucharistic elements is converted into the body and blood of Christ at consecration. In some sub-Saharan African settings a positive answer to the question 'does somebody want to harm you?' does not necessarily mean a paranoid delusion, because it might simply reflect a fear of witchcraft and sorcery.

Hallucinations

When considering the context of hallucinations, cultural factors including religious expectations, ritual, the use of psychoactive substances and the degree of acculturation must all be considered. The practitioner has to ask: 'Are these visions or voices culturally sanctioned?'. Failure to do this can lead to misdiagnosis in people from ethnic minorities.

In patients with schizophrenia in the West, auditory hallucinations are reported roughly twice as frequently as visual hallucinations. Conversely, visual hallucinations are reported more often than auditory hallucinations by patients with schizophrenia in the rest of the world. Historically in the West, visual hallucinations were commoner and were often valorised as communications with God and the saints.

Hallucinations can be part of normal experience with up to one-quarter of the general population in the UK having at least one hallucinatory experience in their lifetime (Slade and Bentall, 1988; Bentall, 2003). Hallucinations might be more commonly experienced in a non-Western cultural setting where the attitude to these perceptions might be very different and they might arouse much less anxiety.

The Western category of hallucination excludes dreams and also makes a rigid distinction between daydreams, imagery and hallucinations. In his research on hallucinations and culture, the psychologist Ihsan Al-Issa (1995) has shown how in some other cultural settings less pathological significance might be attached to these distinctions. On the contrary, hallucinations may be deliberately induced or at least fostered under culturally controlled conditions. The meaning of these intentionally induced hallucinations is shared by the community so they lack psychopathological significance. Far from being evidence of mental illness, the participants in ritually induced altered states of consciousness and trance states in which hallucinations can occur, regard the experience in a positive light, and people might attribute the experience to a privileged contact with the supernatural, e.g. Pentecostals (Littlewood and Lipsedge, 1997).

Al-Issa (1995) helpfully draws attention to the rigid Western materialist categorising of experience into reality and fantasy. Rationalist clinicians conclude that any individual who cannot tell the difference between what they are imagining and the 'real world' is out of touch with reality, and by definition is suffering from a serious mental illness. In other cultural settings 'reality' is used to describe hallucinations, imagery and altered states of consciousness, and people react to these experiences not 'as if' they are real but 'as' real (Al-Issa, 1995, p. 369).

Mrs A was a 40 year old woman from Uganda who was admitted to a general hospital in South London in a delirious state (DSM IV, acute organic psychosyndrome). She had developed a high fever and when unwell and confused she had tried to run away from the medical ward because she could see a giant snake at the end of her bed. After her fever had been controlled by antibiotics and she had become perfectly lucid again, a psychiatrist was asked to see her because she had said that although the 'snake has now gone' she was certain that she had seen one on her bed when she had a high temperature.

The psychiatrist asked Mrs A if she had ever seen a giant snake before. She described how, as a little girl brought up in a remote village, the children were forbidden to go near one part of the river at any time between noon and late afternoon because the bank was haunted by a giant serpent. Mrs A and several of the other village children once dared each other to go to the river bank in the late afternoon. Although they were terrified of being punished, they were excited by their own daring and they crept up to the river, and first one and then each of the children in succession 'saw' the serpent and ran back home in terror. The psychiatrist was reassured by the knowledge that Mrs A's childhood experience had had a 'pathoplastic' effect on the content of her delirium (Weinstein, 1962).

The mainstream rationalist tradition tends to construe certain imaginary experiences in a negative way. They are devalued and dismissed, and people may be ashamed or embarrassed to talk about visions or voices for fear of being labelled as eccentric or insane. Al-Issa (1995) suggests that in a culture where people are encouraged to report their hallucinations, imagery and dreams, because these private events are positively valued and shared, they are actually better equipped to distinguish a morbid, i.e. pathological, hallucination from a benign one than a person brought up in a rationalist culture where *all* non-material experiences tend to be dismissed and stigmatised (Al-Issa, 1995, p. 370).

I believe that it is clinically helpful to try to gauge the understandability of a patient's preoccupations from the perspective of the person's culture and life experiences, both remote and recent. Here is an example of an apparently idiosyncratic set of beliefs and behaviours which Roland Littlewood and I described 25 years ago:

A 40 year old Jamaican woman was brought to hospital by the police after running down the street in her nightdress in the middle of the night, screaming that she was being pursued by giant mushrooms.

Taking into consideration the facts that:

1 she had lost her job because of racial discrimination
2 she had become increasingly sensitive and isolated
3 her house was found to be full of fungi erupting over the wallpaper and there is a popular Caribbean belief that mushrooms are deposited at night by evil spirits (Weinstein, 1962),

we felt that an empathic understanding of her psychotic experiences was possible. The day before her admission under a Section of the Mental Health Act she had had an acrimonious interview with the local housing department, which had rejected her application for rehousing. Her 'psychosis' thus satisfied Jaspers' (1963) criteria for reactivity: an *intelligible* relationship between the *precipitating event* and the *content* of the delusion, together with a *close time relationship* between the two (Littlewood and Lipsedge, 1981).

Culture-bound syndromes

Consider *Negi-Negi* or the wild-man state (Clarke, 1973) described by anthropologists in the New Guinea Highlands.

The principal actor in this drama is a young man who is betrothed to the daughter of a fellow-villager. It is the local custom for the future bridegroom to work in his father-in-law's garden for seven years. Most of the fiancés cope with this obligation but occasionally a young man has a 'breakdown' and 'collapses under the strain', to use the mechanical engineering metaphors of Western fold-psychology. After a short period of brooding and sulking in his house, he rampages through the village, throwing spears and randomly shooting arrows. Nobody actually gets hurt. He charges into his father-in-law's small-holding and tears up the yams and sweet potatoes that he has been carefully cultivating. He is followed around by a crowd of spectators, mainly village children, who call him rude names and throw water or stones at him, but only from a safe distance.

When he is exhausted the wild-man disappears into the forest. After a day or two he returns to the village with no memory whatever of the entire incident (amnesia). Western observers have called this hysteria, while the local explanation is that the young man has been attacked by malevolent spirits which made him behave like a wild pig. The village elders approach the future father-in-law and diplomatically suggest that there should be no further postponement of the wedding so that the spirits that are tormenting the young man can be appeased.

This stereotyped dramatic sequence prompted us to look for Western culture-bound analogues (Littlewood and Lipsedge, 1987).

The most obvious one is non-lethal overdoses in teenage girls and in women, where a similar sequence of events can be identified with a powerless, or thwarted or oppressed person seeking to rectify their situation. After some prodromal signs (e.g. threats of deliberate self-harm) the resentful schoolgirl or the angry woman swallows a handful of Valium or Prozac. She herself calls the ambulance or waits for her feckless partner, who has witnessed the overdose, to dial 999. The scene of this stereotyped drama then shifts to the emergency department of the nearest hospital. After a stomach washout or eating charcoal, the liaison psychiatrists or the deliberate self-harm mental health professional intervenes. The incident will be formulated in biopsychosocial terms and the parents or the male partner will be asked to remove the pressure (which might have been expecting her to take too many A levels or being expected to tolerate the boyfriend's delinquent behaviour, etc).

In both 'wild-man' and non-lethal overdoses there is a triphasic pattern, as in the other dramatic culture-bound syndromes which are really theatrical idioms of distress. There is:

1 a sense of victimhood
2 a more or less public challenge to the cultural norm
3 a resort to the mystical sanction of the spirit world or, in the Western secular world, to the domain of medicine, to rectify the perceived injustice.

'Stress' is the popular and medically fashionable aetiological explanation for such behaviour.

To summarise, the overlap between exotic and Western culture-bound syndromes is as follows:

- short-lived, dramatic, frightening, symbolic inversion of core values
- non-dominant individuals in situations of frustration
- culture-specific, socially learnt patterns of adjusting one's situation by mobilising sympathy or guilt
- resolution by changes in behaviour or expectations of family, partners, line managers, etc
- the individual is not aware/responsible because behaviour is attributed to 'spirit possession' (wild-man) or 'breakdown'/'brain storm'/'disturbed balance of mind' (overdose) (Littlewood and Lipsedge, 1987).

Summary

This chapter has looked at the issue of SEMI in the context of culture, ethnicity and racism. Mental health professionals must work with consideration and sensitivity, and have a responsibility to be culturally informed when providing care and treatment to these potentially vulnerable individuals. It is essential to bear in mind that 'abnormal' in one set of circumstances, culture or country, may be 'normal' and reasonable, in another. Given the firm intellectual grounding of psychiatry in positivism and rationalism, and the dominant English secular ethos, mental health workers have to be vigilant to avoid pathologising religious belief and practice. The need for caution is greatest in the therapeutic encounter with people who adhere to an unfamiliar, innovative or fissiparous group.

Further reading

Bhugra D and Bahl V (eds) (1999) *Ethnicity: an agenda for mental health*. London, Royal College of Psychiatrists: Gaskell Press.

Bhugra D and Bhui K (1997) Cross-cultural psychiatric assessment. *Advances in Psychiatric Treatment* 3:103–10.

Bhugra D and Bhui K (1997) Clinical management of patients across cultures. *Advances in Psychiatric Treatment* 3:233–9.

Bhugra D and Bhui K (1999) Ethnic and cultural factors in psychopharmacology. *Advances in Psychiatric Treatment* 5:89–95.

Bhugra D and Cochrane R (2001) *Psychiatry in Multi-Cultural Britain*. London, Royal College of Psychiatrists: Gaskell Press.

Bhui K (2002) *Racism and Mental Health*. London: Jessica Kingsley.

Bhui K and Bhugra D (2002) Explanatory models for mental distress: implications for clinical practice and research. *British Journal of Psychiatry* 181:6–7.

Dein S and Lipsedge M (1998) Negotiating across culture, race and religion in the inner city. In: Okpaku S (ed.) *Clinical Methods in Transcultural Psychiatry*. Washington, DC: American Psychiatric Association, pp. 137–54.

Fernando S (1995) *Mental Health in a Multi-Ethnic Society: a multi-disciplinary handbook*. London: Routledge.

Fernando S (2005) Multi-cultural mental health services: projects for minority ethnic communities in England. *Transcultural Psychiatry* 42:420–36.

Fernando S, Ndegwa D and Wilson M (1998) *Forensic Psychiatry, Race and Culture*. London: Routledge.

Helman C (2001) *Culture, Health and Illness* (4e). London: Arnold.

Kareem J and Littlewood R (2000) *Intercultural Therapy* (2e). Oxford: Blackwell Science.

Kleinman A (1991) *Rethinking Psychiatry: from cultural category to personal experience*. New York: Free Press.

Laungani P (2004) *Asian Perspectives in Counselling and Psychotherapy*. Hove and New York: Brunner Routledge.

Ndegwa D and Olajide D (eds) (2003) *Main Issues in Mental Health and Race*. Aldershot: Ashgate.

Skultans V (2003) Culture and dialogue in medical psychiatric narratives. *Anthropology and Medicine* 10:155–66.

References

Al-Issa I (1995) The illusion of reality or the reality of illusion: hallucinations and culture. *British Journal of Psychiatry* 166:368–73.

American Psychiatric Association (1994) *DSM IV Diagnostic and Statistical Manual of Mental Disorders* (4e). Washington DC: American Psychiatric Association.

Bentall RP (2003) *Madness Explained: psychosis and human nature*. London: Penguin.

Bhugra D and Ayonrinde O (2001) Racial life events and psychiatric morbidity. In: Bhugra D and Cochrane R (eds) *Psychiatry of Multi-Cultural Britain*. London, Royal College of Psychiatrists: Gaskell Press, pp.91–111.

Bhugra D and Bhui K (1998) Psychotherapy for ethnic minorities: issues context and practice. *British Journal of Psychotherapy* 14:310–26.

Bhugra D and Cochrane R (2001) *Psychiatry in Multi-Cultural Britain*. London, Royal College of Psychiatrists: Gaskell Press.

Bhugra D and Jones P (2001) Migration and mental illness. *Advances in Psychiatric Treatment* 7:216–23.

Bhugra D, Lippett R and Cole E (1999) Pathways into care: an explanation of the factors that may affect minority ethnic groups. In: Bhugra D and Bahl V (eds) *Ethnicity: an agenda for mental health*. London, Royal College of Psychiatrists: Gaskell Press, pp. 29–39.

Boydell J, van Os J, McKenzie K *et al* (2001) Incidence of schizophrenia in ethnic minorities in London: ecological study into interactions with environment. *British Medical Journal* 323:1336–8.

Clarke WC (1973) Temporary madness as theatre: wild-man behaviour in New Guinea. *Oceania* 43:1983–214.

Concise Oxford Dictionary (10e). (2002) Oxford: Oxford University Press.

Coyle BR (2001) Twelve myths of religion and psychiatry: lessons for training psychiatrists in spiritually sensitive treatments. *Mental Health, Religion and Culture* 4:149–74.

Crawford TA and Lipsedge M (2004) Seeking help for psychological distress: the interface of Zulu traditional healing and Western biomedicine. *Mental Health, Religion and Culture* 7:131–48.

Dein S (2002) Moshiach is here now: just open your eyes and you can see him. *Anthropology and Medicine* 9:25–36.

Dein S (2004) *Religion and Healing Among the Lubavitch Community in Stamford Hill, North London: a case study of Hasidism*. Lampeter: The Edwin Mellen Press.

de Jong JTVM and Van Ommeren M (2002) Toward a culture-informed epidemiology: combining qualitative and quantitative research in transcultural contexts. *Transcultural Psychiatry* 39:422–33.

Goldberg D, Bridges K, Duncan-Jones P and Grayson D (1988) Detecting anxiety and depression in general medical settings. *British Medical Journal* 297:897–9.

Harrison JFC (1979) *The Second Coming: popular millenniarism 1780–1850*. London: Routledge and Keegan Paul.

Helman C (2001) *Culture Health and Illness* (4e). London: Arnold.

Heilman SC and Witztum E (2000) All in faith: religion as the idiom and means of coping with distress. *Mental Health, Religion and Culture* 3:115–24.

Hicks JW (2004) Ethnicity, race and forensic psychiatry: are we colour-blind? *Journal of the American Academy of Psychiatry and Law* 32:21–33.

Hussain F and Cochrane R (2004) Depression in South Asian women living in the UK: a review of the literature with implications for service provision. *Transcultural Psychiatry* 41:253–70.

Independent Inquiry into the Death of David Bennett (2003) (Chairman: Sir John Blofeld). Cambridge: Norfolk Suffolk and Cambridgeshire Strategic Health Authority.

Jackson JS, Brown TN, Williams DR *et al* (1996) Racism and the physical and mental health status of African-Americans: a thirteen-year national panel study. *Ethnicity and Disease* 6:132–47.

Jaspers K (1963) *General Psychopathology* (7e, 1958 translation). Manchester: Manchester University Press.

Jenkins J (1998) Diagnostic criteria for schizophrenia and related psychotic disorders: integration and suppression of cultural evidence in DSM-IV. *Transcultural Psychiatry* 35:357–76.

Jenkins JH and Barrett RJ (eds) (2004) *Schizophrenia Culture and Subjectivity*. Cambridge: Cambridge University Press.

Johnson S and Orrell M (1996) Insight psychosis and ethnicity: a case note study. *Psychological Medicine* 26:1081–4.

Kareem J and Littlewood R (2000) *Intercultural Therapy: themes interpretations and practice* (2e). Oxford: Blackwell Scientific Publications.

Kleinman A (1980) *Patients and Healers in the Context of Culture*. Berkley: University of California Press.

Kleinman A (1987) Anthropology and psychiatry: the role of culture in cross cultural research on illness. *British Journal of Psychiatry* 151:447–54.

Kleinman A (1988) *Rethinking Psychiatry: from cultural category to personal experience*. New York: Free Press.

Kleinman A and Good A (eds) (1985) *Culture and Depression: studies in the anthropology and cross-cultural psychiatry of affect and disorder*. Berkley: University of California Press.

Laming L (2003) *The Victoria Climbié Inquiry: presented to Parliament by the Secretary of State for Health and the Secretary of State for the Home Department by command of Her Majesty January 2003*. Cm5730. London: The Stationery Office.

Leyman H (1996) The content and development of mobbing at work. *European Journal of Work and Organisational Psychology* 5:165–84.

Lim RF and Lin KM (1996) Psychosis following *Qi-Gong* in a Chinese immigrant. *Culture, Medicine and Psychiatry* 22:369–78.

Lipsedge M (1994) Dangerous stereotypes. *Journal of Forensic Psychiatry* 5:14–19.

Lipsedge M (2003) Jonathan Martin: prophet and incendiary. *Mental Health, Religion and Culture* 6:59–77.

Littlewood R (1983) The Antinomian Hasid. *British Journal of Medical Psychology* 56:67–78.

Littlewood R (1984) The imitation of madness: the influence of psychopathology. *Culture, Social Science and Medicine* 19:705–15.

Littlewood R and Lipsedge M (1981) Acute psychotic reactions in Caribbean-born patients. *Psychological Medicine* 11:303–18.

Littlewood R and Lipsedge M (1987) The butterfly and the serpent: culture, psychopathology and biomedicine. *Culture, Medicine and Psychiatry* 11:289–335.

Littlewood R and Lipsedge M (1997) *Aliens and Alienists: ethnic minorities and psychiatry* (3e). London: Routledge.

Loewenthal KM (1995) *Religion and Mental Health*. London: Chapman and Hall.

Mason D (2000) *Race and Ethnicity in Modern Britain* (2e). Oxford: Oxford University Press.

Massé ER (2002) *Gadé* deceptions and lies told by the ill: the Caribbean socio-cultural construction of truth in patient–healer encounters. *Anthropology and Medicine* 9:175–88.

Nazroo JY (1997) *Ethnicity and Mental Health: findings from a community survey*. London: Policy Studies Institute.

Pearsall J (ed.) (1998) *The New Oxford Dictionary of English*. Oxford: Oxford University Press.

Ryder AG, Bean G and Dion KL (2000) Caregiver responses to symptoms of first-onset psychosis: a comparative study of Chinese and Euro-Canadian families. *Transcultural Psychiatry* 37:255–65.

Saravanan B, Jacob KS, Prince M, Bhugra D and David AS (2004) Culture and insight revisited. *British Journal of Psychiatry* 184:107–9.

Schmitt R (1996) Racism and objectification. In: Gordon LR, Sharpley-Whiting TD and White RT (eds) *Fanon: a critical reader*. Oxford: Blackwell, pp. 35–52.

Sharma B and Van Ommeren M (1998) Preventing torture and rehabilitating survivors in Nepal. *Transcultural Psychiatry* 35:87–98.

Sims A (1988) *Symptoms in the Mind*. London: Baillière Tindall.

Slade PD and Bentall RP (1988) *Sensory Deception: a scientific analysis of hallucinations*. London: Croom-Helm.

Special Hospital Service Authority (1993) *Report of the Committee of Inquiry into the death at Broadmoor Hospital of Orville Blackwood and a review of the deaths of two other Afro-Caribbean patients. The Prins Report*. London: HMSO.

Spiro AM (2005) *Najar* or *Bhutt:* evil eye or ghost affliction: Gujarati views about illness causation. *Anthropology and Medicine* 12:61–74.

Thomas L (2000) Racism and psychotherapy: working with racism in the consulting room; an analytical view. In: Kareem J and Littlewood R (eds) *Intercultural Therapy: themes, interpretations and practice* (2e). Oxford: Blackwell Scientific Publications, pp. 146–60.

Weinstein EA (1962) *Cultural Aspects of Delusion*. London: Collier-MacMillan.

World Health Organization (1992) *ICD-10. Classification of Mental and Behavioural Disorders*. Geneva: World Health Organization.

Chapter 7

Political and philosophical dimensions of severe and enduring mental illness

Rachel Freeth

If you have a SEMI you could be referred to the PMHT, CMHT, CRHTT or ACTT, via an ICP, ending up with a CPA[1]

Introduction

SEMI (severe and enduring mental illness) is just one of the many acronyms that now liberally sprinkle the daily conversations of NHS health professionals, within an organisation that has become bewilderingly complex and fragmented. In an admittedly exaggerated way, the opening sentence is intended less to highlight the (often irritating) use of acronyms, and more to highlight a prevalent feature of NHS mental healthcare. This is the continual creation of categories of disorder and new teams to which various categories of patients are referred. Alongside increasing categorisation is the development of the 'integrated care pathway' that attempts to set standards for who, what, when and how care is delivered. This situation demonstrates realities that, in my view, deserve closer analysis from a philosophical and political point of view. This chapter aims to offer this.

I am a psychiatrist with an interest in philosophy and an observer of the political scene, particularly concerning healthcare and mental health policy. However, I acknowledge that the topics of both philosophy and politics leave many fellow health professionals either uninterested or distinctly uncomfortable. It is therefore a mark of boldness and open mindedness that the editor of this book wished to include a chapter that will perhaps sit rather awkwardly alongside fellow contributions. Nevertheless, it is my hope that it may offer the reader a useful broader context when thinking about how to respond to people with SEMI in primary care. Much of this chapter is also highly relevant to those working in secondary care.

What I should make clear is that this chapter concerns the category and term 'severe and enduring mental illness', what it means and some of the consequences of its use. It is not about the condition of mental disorder itself such as the philosophical topic of phenomenology of mental disorders. Perhaps I should

---

[1] SEMI – severe and enduring mental illness; PMHT – primary mental health team; CMHT – community mental health team; CRHTT – crisis resolution home treatment team; ACTT – assertive community treatment team; ICP – integrated care pathway; CPA – care programme approach

also declare at the outset that I dislike the term (and the acronym SEMI) and the way it is increasingly used within health settings. While I partly understand why the term has arisen, I regard it as having potentially damaging consequences for patients, as well as being of limited practical use. In highlighting some of these consequences, my intention is to facilitate greater reflective practice and perhaps limit some of the negative effects of using the term. I begin though, with considering the political backdrop against which increasing use of the category severe and enduring mental illness has been strongly influenced.

The era of categorisation: political influences

The increasing gap between public expectations and the supply of services has led policy-makers to consider new ways to ensure that limited resources are used efficiently and more equitably

(Coulter, 2002, p. 100).

As the demand for mental health services has increased over recent years, the resources available within both primary and secondary care have not kept pace to meet those demands that are driven, in part, by increasing public expectations. Services, and the professionals who work in them, have struggled and are increasingly struggling to cope with the volume and complexity of mental health needs presented to them daily.

When the current Labour Government came to power in 1997, it set about addressing the problems bedevilling the NHS, caused partly by years of gross under-funding. To this end it formulated the ambitious *NHS Plan* (Department of Health, 2000). In recognition that the mental health service was one of the areas that needed particular attention it also produced the *National Service Framework* (NSF) *for Mental Health* (Department of Health, 1999). This massive programme of reform within mental health services has continued to gather pace ever since, with a constant stream of new policies and guidance flowing from the Department of Health. One of the legacies of this government has been the firm establishment of a healthcare culture that demonstrates a 'rigorous pursuit of efficiency and cost-effectiveness' (Department of Health, 1998, p. 64), that strives to achieve 'key deliverables' (pursues targets), is evidence based and 'outcome driven', and which is influenced by the principles of a market economy and uses competition as the basis of motivation to provide more efficient and effective services.

A health system that seeks to be efficient and cost-effective with its limited resources needs to ask two key questions: first, to which people, or group of patients, should health services be targeting its resources, i.e. who, or which type of problem, is eligible for help? Secondly, which part of the service, or group of professionals, treats which problems? Given that in the UK a clear feature of healthcare provision is the division between primary and secondary care, this second question could translate to which patients can or should be treated in primary care and which in secondary care? Primary care has the more comprehensive picture of mental health needs in the community and it therefore makes sense for the initial assessment and screening of mental health needs to take place within primary care settings, which can thereby also act as the gatekeeper to specialist secondary mental health care resources.

Primary care is currently facing the enormous challenge of how best to meet the needs of people who are variously described as experiencing mental distress, have mental health problems or who have a mental illness. Not only is responding to mental distress often very emotionally demanding work in itself, but GPs can find it difficult to access specialist help. Some of these difficulties include knowing who to ask for help and how to make a referral. Furthermore, because mental health needs have to be prioritised, it is difficult to know the threshold for making a specialist referral and how to decide whether the referral is routine or urgent. What should help in addressing these issues, especially as GPs vary hugely in their training and experience in dealing with psychological and psychiatric issues in patients, is the development of specialist mental health workers within primary care. These are the so-called 'gateway workers', one of whose functions is to co-ordinate access to specialist secondary care services, as well as develop and support mental healthcare within the primary care setting (Department of Health, 2002a). However, it is relatively early days for the development of this new role, and not all GP practices have the benefit of these professionals providing an interface between primary and secondary care.

The existence of gateway workers is clear evidence of the shift towards a primary care-led NHS. The *NSF for Mental Health* laid down standards that included the need for primary care to develop its resources, which would include developing assessment and referral procedures. The future structure of mental health services within primary care and secondary care is now very much dependent on what primary care trusts (PCTs) decide is needed, although the government has already stipulated certain 'must haves' such as 24-hour crisis resolution home treatment teams. It is PCTs that will largely influence the structure and role of specialist mental health services through the process of commissioning services. Practice-based commissioning is to be rolled out across all general practices in the NHS in England. Commissioning strategies determine priorities of care provision and the mechanisms and processes by which specialist mental healthcare is accessed and managed. In other words, PCTs are deciding which models of service provision to use when meeting the mental health needs of patients within primary care, which includes deciding which specialist secondary care services they want and most need. Decisions are also being made about which models of mental health services to develop within primary care settings, although there is very little evidence as to which systems are the most effective (Bower and Gilbody, 2005). It is also likely that decisions will be influenced according to cost, and which system is thought likely to save the most money in the short term. In summary then, PCTs are now 'accountable for commissioning cost-effective evidence-based care in accordance with national standards aiming to benefit patient care' (Aitken and Tylee, 2001, p. 459). They are charged with the responsibility for assessing health needs in the local community and for designing a system to which there is a clear point of access and through which a patient travels in the smoothest, most efficient and cost-effective way.

What I hope I am demonstrating is that in the minds of those redesigning services and shaping policy and guidance, there is a need for clarity about roles, functions and responsibilities of different health professionals and of all the various teams within the service. There is a need, for example, for clearer boundaries of responsibility between primary and secondary care for patients with mental health needs. Currently these boundaries are often blurred, creating confusion and tensions in the relationships of health professionals, such as those between GPs and psychiatrists. Many GPs see their responsibility principally for providing the physical care of patients with mental health problems, whereas others take a far more active and direct role in providing mental healthcare.

Another increasingly dominant feature of healthcare culture is the focus on clearly defined goals and outcomes. In the minds of managers and politicians, these outcomes should ideally be measurable. There is also increasing interest in recording and measuring the activities of professionals working towards specified goals. The more short-term and focused the intervention the better. Ultimately, the aim seems to be for all care to be translated somehow into numerical terms and therefore cost. The government aims to set national tariffs for all interventions that will be linked to specific predicted outcomes. This is the basis on which 'payment by results' will operate (Department of Health, 2002b). This is a new method of paying for both hospital and community health services in which care providers will be paid according to quantity of work and specific outcomes. The intention is for competition between providers to drive up efficiency and increase motivation.

To enable the development and operation of a healthcare organisation as described above, it becomes necessary for a certain process to occur. This is the process of *categorisation*. In this context, categorisation involves defining types of patients and their mental health needs according to objective criteria, in order to determine what to do for them, or with them. The aim is to achieve a more standardised, and therefore more easily measurable and costable, response and treatment, according to the category of problem or need. What has emerged is the notion that there are broadly two categories of mental disorders generally known in the literature as 'common mental health problems' and 'severe and enduring mental illness'.

Difficulties defining severe and enduring mental illness

Attempts to define SEMI are not new. In 1996, following the inquiry into the care and treatment of Christopher Clunis, the Department of Health published *Building Bridges*, which was guidance to promote co-ordinated care and more effective inter-agency working for severely mentally ill people (Department of Health, 1996). It was decided that services needed to focus their efforts and resources on severely mentally ill people, but in order to do this there would be a need for clarity as to which people should be targeted and prioritised, which meant defining 'severe mental illness'. It was acknowledged that thus far there was no universally agreed definition. A 'framework definition' was therefore offered, focusing on the three recognised dimensions of severe mental illness, namely, diagnosis, disability and duration. Two other dimensions were added, these being safety to self and others and the presence of formal or informal care. However, this makes the definition so broad, and, with no suggestion as to weighting of these dimensions, operationally useless.

Regarding the criterion of diagnosis, severely mentally ill people were seen as 'typically people suffering from schizophrenia or a severe affective disorder, but including dementia' (Department of Health, 1996, p. 11). However, this guidance also seemed to include severe neurotic conditions, personality disorder and developmental disorder. This contrasts with more recently published guidance from The Sainsbury Centre for Mental Health. In *The Primary Care Guide to Managing Severe Mental Illness* (Cohen *et al*, 2004), it is recommended that defining severe mental illness be restricted to only schizophrenia and bipolar affective disorder, the rationale for this being the practical one of making it simpler to create a register of patients with SEMI within general practices. What is certainly apparent from this later guidance and from my own experience, is how much the specific diagnosis is used as the main criterion for defining severe mental illness, even though there remains no clear consensus as to which diagnoses to include.

Another definition of SEMI is provided by Ryan and Pritchard who described it as 'any mental illness that is extremely disabling through its symptoms or its consequences which is long-lasting' (Ryan and Pritchard, 2004). This, too, is extremely broad.

What of duration of illness and the 'enduring' aspect of severe and enduring mental illness? Given how 'severe mental illness' and 'severe and enduring mental illness' are often used interchangeably, for example in the *NSF for Mental Health*, the picture becomes quite confusing. Using the terms interchangeably seems to imply that severe also means enduring. However, the NSF divides severe mental illness into both severe and short-term conditions that can be managed solely within primary care, and severe and enduring conditions where there may be complex needs requiring the input of many agencies such as secondary care services. I may be being pedantic, but I actually think clarity is important here because 'enduring' is not a casual add-on. Illnesses that can endure raise many issues, both practical and emotional. Practical issues may include which social care packages, accommodation or benefits are required and which services should be involved in providing care.

Difficulty also lies in trying to define objectively aspects of conditions that are also highly subjective, such as severity, duration and levels of disability. By what criteria is a condition severe? At what point along the mild, moderate, severe continuum does a condition move into the severe end? When does a condition become enduring? What constitutes extreme disability? Most importantly, who should decide – professionals, mental health services, or patients? Doesn't level of disability depend upon the social context and to a large extent upon patients' and society's perceptions of what the patient can do and in what way they are limited? The attempt to be objective about what is subjective is, in my view, one of the major flaws in using the category severe and enduring mental illness. In practice though, it tends to be the diagnosis that determines whether the illness is considered enduring.

Another objection is the implication in the NSF that the so-called common mental health problems such as depression and anxiety, the other major category, are less severe. Yet depression in some individuals is severe enough to be life-threatening. Just because a condition is common does not mean it cannot be severe and enduring. The use of categories like SEMI and common mental health problems is therefore clearly misleading.

Furthermore, if the rationale for using such categories is to decide more easily which conditions should be treated in primary care and which in secondary care, in my view it fails. Depression, anxiety or eating disorder could be categorised as common conditions, or severe ones requiring the specialist skills one is more likely to find within secondary care services. Severity and disability depend on a range of other factors associated with the individual's personality, relationships and social circumstances. Therefore, deciding which conditions belong to which category on the basis of diagnosis is clearly flawed. Contrary to the prevailing view, psychiatric diagnosis is not a predictor of severity, duration, complexity, risk, or what type of help is likely to be useful.

Diagnosis and the dominance of the medical model

Assessment and diagnosis involve gathering and then ordering (categorising) information. The medical model of assessment, diagnosis and treatment is the predominant model health professionals use within the NHS, particularly the medical profession. What follows are a few comments on the limitations of the medical model, and indeed, its potential harm (explored further in Freeth, 2007). Philosophically, and in practice, I struggle with the medical model as used in psychiatry. Unsurprisingly, this makes my working life as a psychiatrist fraught with tensions.

Primarily, I view the medical model as a particular activity and method of working that has a major influence on the nature of the relationship between the patient and healthcare professional. It usually relies on the expertise of the healthcare professional rather than the patient, and can therefore create a culture of dependency. It can depersonalise people by the tendency to see only the problem to be diagnosed, or in psychiatry, the person to be diagnosed and labelled. The medical model can be exploited as a way of gaining power and has the potential to be abusive and coercive. All of this may interfere with the development of a helpful therapeutic relationship in which the patient also significantly contributes to the process.

The medical model uses the language of illness, pathology (psychopathology) and dysfunction. It focuses on symptoms and their treatment rather than attending to the whole person. The medical model reinforces a reductionist rather than holistic approach, reductionism being the process of taking things apart and reducing them down to the simplest level to study them. The reliance on the medical model within psychiatry also illustrates the dominance of the paradigm known by philosophers as logical positivism. This is a paradigm based on objective observation and which is mechanistic. It has had a major influence on the neurosciences and the development of cognitive and behavioural psychology. Positivism underlies most of the quantitative research that is regarded as the 'gold standard', such as randomised controlled trials. Indeed, the popularity of cognitive-behavioural therapy within mental health services (and cognitive-behavioural approaches to mental health generally), illustrates just how dominant objectivity and logical positivism are within our culture, indicating the psychological need, and therefore quest, for certainty in an uncertain and unpredictable world.

What I challenge is not science and logical positivism themselves, since they have contributed vastly to our understanding of the natural world, but their dominance within psychiatry at the expense of other paradigms and approaches. Currently relatively little attention is paid to approaches that focus on values and meaning or on existential issues in which the patient's subjective experience is attended to, without the need to explain or interpret it. Approaches that champion objectivity, and that are symptom orientated, rely on explanatory frameworks which often reinforce disease theories of mental disorder, i.e. that mental disorder has a physical, organic cause, with the biochemical imbalance theory being the most popular.

Diagnosis, an inherent part of the medical model, is an aspect of psychiatry I am increasingly uncomfortable with. I challenge the way in which diagnostic categories group individuals and their symptoms, or symptom clusters, in order to predict, for example, the natural course of a disorder and prognosis following specific treatments. While I can see some value in the recognition of commonalities and patterns where they exist (and for many patients it can be valuable knowing fellow sufferers with the same diagnosis, reducing a sense of isolation), there is also a clear danger of ignoring the uniqueness of individuals, including their personalities and circumstances.

Despite the rhetoric of government promising an NHS that shapes 'its services around the needs and preferences of individual patients, their families and their carers' (Department of Health, 2000), in reality treatment and management have become more standardised and 'manualised' and not tailored to the individual. It is here I want to turn my attention to the integrated care pathway (sometimes known as the clinical pathway, care map or pathway of care).

The development and proliferation of integrated care pathways, which I shall from here simply refer to as the care pathway, are now dominant features of NHS care. Since their development from the early 1990s, care pathways have provided a clear illustration and evidence of the underlying values and philosophy of modern day healthcare. Often depicted by an algorithm or flow chart, care pathways aim to detail the various stages of care patients may experience. They chart the patient's journey through the healthcare system, highlighting each intervention, who it was by and at what point in time. They enable the structuring of the process of care into a describable sequence of steps.

Advocates of care pathways point to how they may enable greater planning of care and how they can support the use of clinical guidelines, the implementation of protocols and better co-ordination of care. Whatever the merits from a clinical point of view though, these are nothing compared to what they offer managers, for care pathways are the ultimate efficiency tool enabling tighter management of resources. Through the creation of streamlined and standardised episodes of care, care pathways offer a method of controlling the patient's journey as he or she 'flows' through the system.

However, I do not find it hard to see patients moving around the NHS system as analogous to products being processed around different sections of the factory floor in predetermined sequences and time-frames with the expected progress and outcomes that are the result of quantitative evidence-based research. Care pathways might work for Mr and Mrs 'typical and predictable' (who I don't think I have ever met yet), but not for Mr and Mrs 'unique', who require an individual approach to care and who would prefer to be treated as persons rather than as products with commercial value. Furthermore, care pathways remove from the equation one vital variable of care – the nature of the relationship between health professional and patient. It is for this reason that care pathways, in my view, are not only flawed but potentially harmful in not emphasising the importance and value of relationship in care, particularly mental healthcare.

Disorder-specific treatments are another outcome of diagnosis-driven (or category-driven) mental healthcare. The development of dialectical behaviour therapy for people diagnosed with borderline personality disorder (Linehan, 1993; Palmer, 2002) is a good recent example. Yet diagnosis alone is, in my view, a poor way of deciding treatment because, like care pathways, it doesn't take into account a person's social circumstances, attitudes, personality traits and a host of other variables that affect treatment outcomes. This is one of many reasons for questioning the validity of diagnosis, not to mention the highly questionable reliability of psychodiagnosis.

While SEMI is not in itself a diagnostic category such as those categories of mental disorder listed in the *International Classification of Disease* (ICD-10, World Health Organization, 1992) and the *Diagnostic and Statistical Manual of Mental Disorders* (DSM-IV, American Psychiatric Association, 1994), it has many of the features of diagnosis in terms of its application and how people think and behave in relation to it.

The language of diagnosis risks stereotyping, with the tendency to think that 'schizophrenics need this', 'borderliners do that' and 'somatisers[2] behave in this way'. Such stereotyping could become magnified with the use of the category SEMI, and many of these stereotypes are negative as a result of the association of mental illness with violence and dangerousness, certainly in the minds of an often ignorant public and media. With the government's preoccupation with public safety and controlling risk, this becomes yet another group of individuals to observe and control. This excessive and neurotic preoccupation is, in my opinion, one of the more disturbing outcomes of a risk-management culture. This must be one of the main reasons why the *NSF for Mental Health* gives higher priority to people with severe mental illnesses. Unfortunately, this ensures that others with high levels of morbidity, such as people with profoundly disturbed personalities, or those who misuse substances, get a raw deal in terms of the distribution of healthcare resources.

Treatment and recovery

Regarding the treatment of SEMI (notice the depersonalisation and narrow focus of this statement), another adverse effect of using this category is the risk of stereotyping people as having limited recovery potential. Placing such limits on recovery will undoubtedly influence approaches to treatment and management. Beliefs about prognosis will influence attitudes towards what interventions might be worthwhile and cost-effective. Given that enduring generally means permanent, people with a SEMI may as a result be considered not worth the investment of time and effort in providing healthcare. The implication of SEMI is that diagnosis and disability are for life. Given that for schizophrenia 25–30% of individuals make a complete recovery (return to premorbid functioning with no further episodes of illness)[3], it is clearly false to regard schizophrenia, one of

---

[2] Borderliners – patients diagnosed with borderline personality disorder; somatisers – patients diagnosed with somatisation disorder, who are thought to express psychological problems through physical symptoms

[3] Web sources quoting these figures include the National Institute for Mental Health in England and the charity RETHINK (previously known as National Schizophrenia Fellowship)

the diagnoses placed in this category, as enduring for everyone given this diagnosis. Furthermore, even though the presence of certain factors may predispose to a good or poor prognosis, there is no way of reliably predicting the prognosis of schizophrenia for any individual. Nevertheless, mental health professionals continue to make predictions about recovery. Might such false predictions occur less often without the category of SEMI?

One of the factors that is likely to influence the course of mental illness and recovery is what support and treatment are available from primary and secondary care, as well as societal contributions and influences. Decisions around which services and treatments to provide are those considered most cost-effective and validated by evidence-based research. Such research usually relies on a biomedical view of illness. Severity of illness is measured, often via rating scales and scoring systems that focus on symptoms and specific deficits. In the medical model, treatment is administered by the health professional to reduce or eradicate symptoms. What is often absent when considering which services to provide and approaches to use, is a language of healing, growth, human potentials, spiritual dimensions and essentially all those many aspects of being human that cannot be measured and that are not amenable to the current forms of evidence-based research. This is as much the case for SEMI as for other mental disturbances. In my view this is a narrow and grossly short-sighted approach to helping people with mental disturbance, of whatever form and however severe.

What I observe is a lack of consideration and attention to relationship (including, crucially, relationships with professionals and other helpers) and environmental influences. It is these that, in my view, contribute significantly to mental wellbeing, growth and recovery. Because this is not easily translated into measurable outcomes, approaches that emphasise these factors are easily dismissed (in practice if not in theory) because the quantitative evidence cannot be provided.

Most people with a SEMI will be prescribed psychotropic medication, while the general perception is that counselling and psychotherapy are unsuitable for SEMI, unless they use cognitive-behavioural approaches (*see* Freeth 2004 for a discussion on the uses of psychotropic drugs, influences on prescribing and debates surrounding their use, especially in relation to counselling and psychotherapy). Counselling tends to be viewed as an ineffective treatment, although this is not proven because the research is lacking. However, cognitive-behavioural therapy and medication are well ahead in terms of evidence-based research, and this is precisely what commissioners of services will be looking for.

The other issue for counselling and psychotherapy is the fact that many approaches, for example the person-centred approach, do not regard themselves as a treatment in terms of the medical model, i.e. to remove symptoms or work towards measurable goals. Rather, counselling and psychotherapy 'provide a unique opportunity for the client or patient to be offered time and attention . . . In this context they are not considered a diagnosis, a "problem", or merely a service user. The person is truly met as a "person" . . .' (Eatock and Russello, 2004). In other words the aim of counselling and psychotherapy is quite different from usual psychiatric interventions. The person-centred approach in particular offers a relationship and therapeutic climate that aim to enable the person to find their own resources and move towards growth and healing, while also being less likely to encourage the dependency that traditional psychiatric approaches tend to do. Furthermore, the person-centred approach is not diagnosis specific, and is therefore suitable for people with SEMI, as long as individual counsellors and psychotherapists are comfortable and confident in knowing their limitations where these exist. The person-centred approach has also developed a method of working called pre-therapy for people who have impaired psychological contact, such as those with psychosis, dissociation or dementia (Prouty *et al*, 2002).

Finally, in my experience, counselling and psychotherapy can work well with the so-called 'recovery model' of mental illness, albeit perhaps needing to adopt greater flexibility of boundaries and attention to the environment. The concept of recovery reflects values-based practice rather than evidence-based practice, promotes a holistic approach and attempts to be user led and focuses on a person's strengths and assets rather than their deficits. There is much here that many counsellors and psychotherapists will recognise as important. Their contribution to the recovery of people with SEMI is, in my opinion, invaluable.

A good example of a long-term counselling relationship with someone given a diagnosis of paranoid schizophrenia is provided by Brown (2004), who also asserts that the motivation and commitment of the client are more reliable indicators of therapeutic change than diagnosis.

Financial considerations

Diagnosis is increasingly the basis on which health services are organised and funded, as highlighted earlier. One of the big risks of a diagnosis-driven health system and the proposed funding arrangement of 'payment by results', is the manipulation of diagnosis for financial gain, particularly in a cost-conscious and cash-strapped organisation. Within general practice, the category of SEMI offers an opportunity for receiving extra payments through providing enhanced services as part of the *New General Medical Services* (GMS) *Contract* for GPs (NHS Confederation and British Medical Association, 2003).

One of the reasons for compiling a register of people with SEMI, as mentioned earlier, is to provide annual physical health checks for this group of patients. It is of course only right that the physical needs of these patients should be identified given that, according to research, the physical health of people with schizophrenia and bipolar affective disorder is significantly poorer than that of comparative groups without these illnesses (Cohen *et al*, 2004). This is why it is recommended that this category be restricted to these two diagnoses only. Yet, what about the physical health needs of people with other diagnoses? Emphasis on a particular group may lead to relative neglect of other groups.

However, my main objection concerns the underlying financial motivation. Creating a register is worth a certain number of points, and points mean payments. In the new GMS contract mental health is worth a certain number of points. Of all the points available for mental healthcare, most are for SEMI. Regrettably, this ignores the vast amount of work GPs do managing other forms of mental distress.

Potentially, a diagnosis becomes equated with various sizes of payments and the risks of this happening increase if 'payment by results' takes hold of health services. Interventions and treatments may also be manipulated because of what they cost or earn, depending on who is buying or selling services. It is hard to see, though, how this system can be applied to people with SEMI, given the complexity and diversity of needs these people often have. Furthermore, SEMI does not lend itself to the 'robust' classification system 'payment by results' relies upon.

Conclusion

The category and term severe and enduring mental illness open up many issues and debates which are frequently either swept under the carpet or blurred, either deliberately or unwittingly. These are complex areas that are difficult to think about. Discussing them is additionally difficult because they challenge a culture in which there are vested interests of a personal, professional, financial and political nature to keep things as they are. Challenging paradigms is difficult. While one definition of a paradigm is 'a constellation of shared assumptions, beliefs and values' (Okasha, 2002, p. 81), paradigms have also been described as 'whole systems of prejudice' (Ingleby, 1980, p. 25). Ingleby also says that 'negotiation between the holders of different paradigms is difficult, not only because each paradigm uses a different conceptual system, but because each represents different *interests*' (Ingleby, 1980, p. 26, original italics). When paradigms are driven by political and economic interests, it is hard not to be powerfully influenced by them. It becomes difficult, if not impossible, not to speak the language of the system within which one works. Not to do so would risk alienation.

What I hope this chapter achieves is at least to make practitioners more aware of what underlies the language and terminology they use and what attitudes language is capable of perpetuating. The category of SEMI tells us many things about the health culture in which we work and from which we receive care. It tells us many things about the structure of, and policies within, mental health services. And while it may have its uses, there is, in my view, a heavy cost involved. The mental health service is becoming increasingly mechanised and professionals more like technicians. I believe there is a fundamental loss of human values within an organisation driven by a business ethic and economic values that places severe constraints on cultivating vital healing relationships. This is a mental health system (and health system in general) that is becoming ever more dehumanising for both patients and staff. It could be pointed out that at least we no longer have the enormous asylums in which people were incarcerated for the most preposterous of reasons, but today's dehumanising activities are perhaps equally sinister because they are less overt.

My desire is for a mental health service in which humanistic attitudes and values have a significant influence. O'Hara writes:

> *Contemporary culture desperately needs a coherent shared vision. Part of that need is for a new psychology of wellness, of the sacred, and of empowerment; a psychology that gives meaning and significance to individual human lives, that understands the central importance of stable families and communities, and that can make room for diversity, commonality, and the possibilities for significant connections among us*

(O'Hara, 1997, p. 28).

I share her emancipatory vision and I am concerned that the category of SEMI greatly hinders working towards such a vision.

Acknowledgements

My thanks to Phill Morgan-Henshaw and Peter Smith for their comments on an early draft; also to April Russello for giving me this opportunity to develop and clarify my own thinking and understanding.

References

Aitken P and Tylee A (2001) The future of primary care groups and mental health commissioning. *Psychiatric Bulletin* 25:459–61.

American Psychiatric Association (1994) *Diagnostic and Statistical Manual of Mental Disorders* (4e). Washington DC: American Psychiatric Association.

Bower P and Gilbody S (2005) Managing common mental health disorders in primary care: conceptual models and evidence. *British Medical Journal* 330:839–42.

Brown M (2004) Long-term counselling for someone with paranoid schizophrenia. *Healthcare Counselling and Psychotherapy Journal* 4:6–9.

Coulter A (2002) *The Autonomous Patient. Ending paternalism in medical care.* London: The Nuffield Trust.

Cohen A, Singh SP and Hague J (2004) *The Primary Care Guide to Managing Severe Mental Illness.* London: The Sainsbury Centre for Mental Health.

Department of Health (1996) *Building Bridges. A guide to arrangements for inter-agency working for the care and protection of severely mentally ill people.* London: Department of Health.

Department of Health (1998) *Modernising Mental Health Services. Safe, sound and supportive.* London: Department of Health.

Department of Health (1999) *A National Service Framework for Mental Health.* London: Department of Health.

Department of Health (2000) *The NHS Plan. A plan for investment. A plan for reform.* London: Department of Health.

Department of Health (2002a) *Fast-Forwarding Primary Care Mental Health: 'Gateway' Workers.* London: Department of Health.

Department of Health (2002b) *Reforming NHS Financial Flows: Introducing Payment by Results.* London: Department of Health.

Eatock J and Russello A (2004) The distinctive contribution of counselling/psychotherapy to health and healthcare in Britain. *Healthcare Counselling and Psychotherapy Journal* 4:2–3.

Freeth R (2004) *Psychopharmacology, and Counselling and Psychotherapy.* Information Sheet for the British Association for Counselling and Psychotherapy (BACP). Rugby: British Association for Counselling and Psychotherapy.

Freeth R (2007) *Humanising Psychiatry and Mental Health Care. The challenge of the person-centred approach.* Oxford: Radcliffe Publishing.

Ingleby D (1980) *Critical Psychiatry. The politics of mental health.* London: Free Association Books.

Linehan M (1993) *Cognitive-behavioural Treatment of Borderline Personality Disorder.* New York: Guilford Press.

NHS Confederation and British Medical Association (2003) *New General Medical Services Contract 2003 – Investing in General Practice.* London: NHS Confederation and British Medical Association.

O'Hara M (1997) Emancipatory therapeutic practice in a turbulent transmodern era: a work of retrieval. *Journal of Humanistic Psychology* 37:7–33.

Okasha S (2002) *Philosophy of Science.* Oxford: Oxford University Press.

Palmer R (2002) Dialectical behaviour therapy for borderline personality disorder. *Advances in Psychiatric Treatment* 8:10–16.

Prouty G, Van Werde D and Pörtner M (2002) *Pre-Therapy. Reaching contact-impaired clients.* Ross-on-Wye: PCCS Books.

Ryan T and Pritchard J (2004) Preface. In: Ryan T and Pritchard J (eds) *Good Practice in Adult Mental Health.* London: Jessica Kingsley Publishers, pp. 11–12.

World Health Organization (1992) *International Classification of Disease* (10e). Geneva: World Health Organization.

Chapter 8

The association between pain and mental ill-health

Michael Harris

Introduction

Pain is a most common feature of bodily illness and is a *purely psychological phenomenon* (Kendell, 2001). Although actual tissue damage is detected by the nervous system (nociception), the perception of this as pain is a conscious experience, usually resulting in suffering – an emotional experience. This emotional experience appears to be altered and influenced by psychosocial factors, that is, by factors other than the tissue damage itself (Raja and Dougherty, 2005). Armed with this information, one can begin to see why pain is relevant to mental health.

On a mundane level, most of us have had the experience of those psychosocial factors that may alter our pain perception, both in a negative and a positive direction. During a trivial viral illness such as a cold or influenza, or during a particularly stressful period of time, pain from a previous back strain, for example, may seem particularly intense. On the other hand, in the midst of a happy occasion with family or friends, we may dance on an ankle which was sprained only days ago, without apparent regard to the discomfort.

Numerous research studies confirm this link between mood and physical symptoms of pain or discomfort. An American study reports the presence of physical manifestations of discomfort in 70% to 80% of patients with significant symptoms of depression. In most cases those physical symptoms were actually the symptoms first presented to the physician by the patient (Kirkmayer *et al*, 1993). In another study, the presence and number of physical symptoms in primary care patients increased the likelihood of an anxiety or depressive disorder being present in those patients. The greater the number of uncomfortable physical symptoms, the greater the rate of anxiety and depressive disorder, measured by validated questionnaires, and also the greater degree of functional impairment (Kroenke *et al*, 1994). Counsellors and other healthcare practitioners may well find themselves working with such individuals, and knowledge of the impact that pain may have can help facilitate empathy and help make sense of the association between pain and mental ill-health.

Sometimes a specific type of physical symptom appears linked to a specific type of emotional or mental health disorder. A Scandinavian study shows a high prevalence of musculoskeletal pain, with reduced musculoskeletal functioning, in depressive patients (Hallstrom and Posse, 1998).

In order to explain the link between the physical and the mental with regard to pain, it is helpful to understand something of the anatomy, physiology and chemistry of pain. This will now be briefly outlined.

Pain pathways and physiology

Unlike the senses (such as sight or hearing), in which specific receptors are stimulated by the factor to be detected (e.g. a light image falling upon the nerve cells in the retina of the eye; sound waves setting up vibrations within the ear and causing stimulation of the auditory nerves) there are *no* specific pain receptors. Rather, it is chemical or physical stimulation (or over-stimulation) of nerve endings used for detecting other modalities, such as heat, touch, pressure, which initiate the nerve impulses eventually perceived as pain.

The nerve impulses produced by these stimuli are then *transmitted* along several possible nerve pathways in the peripheral nerves and the spinal cord.

Upon entering the spinal cord (in the dorsal horn) the nerve fibres make connections with other nerve fibres arranged in layers or laminae, before proceeding up the spinal cord (in the dorsal columns, or in the spinoreticular tracts) and eventually terminating in various separate but interconnected centres in the brain.

The impulses are usually *modulated* on their way to these brain centres in various possible ways. Within the spinal cord ordinary stimuli from A-beta fibres may inhibit or block the noxious impulses being carried in A-delta or C fibres, reducing the transmission of impulses which would lead to pain. This (the so-called Gate Control Theory) can explain how scratching or rubbing a painful part of the body can actually reduce the pain. The theory also partly explains the effectiveness of acupuncture and transcutaneous electrical nerve stimulation (TENS) machines as pain treatments.

Modulation can also enhance the painful stimulus. In the 'wind-up' phenomenon, the C-fibre activity is progressively increased by spinal or central activity from above, so that nerve cells become more sensitive to the painful stimulus. This can explain why sufferers of chronic pain often respond to mild touch in a way which seems an exaggerated pain response. They are not being histrionic, nor are they necessarily malingering. Their nervous system, through the adaptive process known as *neuronal plasticity*, has become sensitised to pain.

Brain centres and interconnections of the pain pathways are complex and incompletely understood. Numerous sites have been identified in the cortex, neocortex, medulla and mid-brain, thalamus and hypothalamus, and reticular activating system. It is of interest that these various centres take part in: identifying the pain location (sensory cortex); producing a motor response, such as a gasp or cry or withdrawal of the endangered part of the body (motor cortex); producing an increase in respiration, heart rate, pupil dilatation (midbrain and hypothalamic centres); influence upon general alertness (reticular-activating system); and – most relevant to the topic of this chapter – the overlay of the emotional responses of suffering, anxiety, and depressed mood (the limbic system) which comprise the pain perception.

It is also of interest that the chemical transmitters that convey the impulses between nerve connections in these central pathways (opioids, GABA, norepinephrine (noradrenaline), serotonin – to name only a few) are also known to affect mood. This, in fact, provides the theoretical basis for the use of many medications for mental health, such as antidepressants.

It can be seen, therefore, that the appreciation of pain and emotional lack of wellbeing are intimately entwined. They share similar neuronal pathways, brain centres and chemistry.

(Most of the above section was from Benzon *et al*, 2005.)

Somatisation

The above explains how a physical trauma, producing actual or threatened tissue damage, is translated into the unpleasant experience of pain. In many cases, however, especially in the field of mental health, no physical cause of the pain can be identified.

This is known as somatisation. Many syndromes of 'somatoform disorders' have been described, but as a concept, somatisation is the association of physical symptoms with psychological distress (Kendell and Zealley, 1994). Put another way, somatisation is a process by which a psychiatric disorder presents in a non-psychiatric setting as medically unexplained physical symptoms (Kamaldeep *et al*, 2002), usually involving very real pain or discomfort.

Somatisation is a very common process. Many of us, in everyday life, may recall having suffered a headache or a stomach pain when we were upset about something, or under pressure to meet some deadline. Epidemiological studies in the US show that the prevalence of somatisation is between 0.03% and 0.4% of the US population. In a series of referrals to a cardiology department, 64% were found to have no detectable physical problem. Females are more prone than males to display somatisation symptoms. The female to male ratio has been measured as 20:1. Sufferers of certain associated syndromes also appear to be at high risk, such as those with irritable bowel syndrome, chronic fatigue syndrome or facial pain syndromes. Indeed, those syndromes are controversial, being regarded by some as examples of somatisation in themselves (Creed *et al*, 1992).

Somatisation is also seen to occur more often amongst the elderly, those living alone and those suffering from a known mental health disorder, particularly anxiety or depression, and there may be cultural factors, the process appearing more prevalent in Indian and Chinese subjects (Green, 2003).

In order that the mental health worker may understand further about the link between pain and psychological wellbeing, it is useful to look at patterns of somatisation in more detail. This can be considered both from the point of view of the symptoms, and from the point of view of the mental health diagnoses or disorders.

Patterns of somatisation according to symptoms

Headache, whether of a migraine or non-migraine type, is a very common symptom in somatisation, leading to numerous referrals to neurological departments in order to exclude a serious condition such as a brain tumour. In Norway, a whole town of 92 500 inhabitants was surveyed for the prevalence of headaches. Subjects who took part (64 500) were also asked to complete rating scales for both anxiety and depression. There was a high correlation between headaches and anxiety, and also a strong correlation, but less so, with depression (Zwart *et al*, 2003). High frequency of headaches, rather than severity, appeared to be the important correlating factor.

Chest pain is also a common presentation. As mentioned above, a high proportion of those referred to a cardiology department in the US exhibited somatisation. In a Turkish study, a series of patients presenting to a cardiology department, but in whom no cause for the pain could be found, were surveyed using the Hospital Anxiety and Depression Scale. Around one-third were found to have high scores, and psychiatric interviews were carried out to establish which of those had a serious anxiety disorder. Of the anxiety disorders, 91% had severe chest pain, and 78% had been admitted for observation in a cardiac unit on previous occasions (Demiryoguran *et al*, 2006).

This would appear to confirm the everyday observation of the anxious individual clutching or patting his/her chest. Speculation upon the meaning of the symptom is risky. However it is tempting to believe that the subject is attempting to relieve a metaphorical heartache.

Mentioned in the introduction of this chapter is the association between musculoskeletal pain and depression. This includes a range of muscle, joint and other skeletal discomfort, including fibromyalgia, a chronic myofascial pain syndrome. Non-specific low back pain in particular, has been thought to predispose patients to depression, but this may not be specific, since the predisposition is no more so than for other chronic medical diseases such as renal failure (Cheatle *et al*, 1990).

Jaw and facial pain (related to dysfunction of the temporomandibular joint) is a common finding among patients with psychiatric disorders. Again, anxiety and depression are the common mental health findings, and again the symptom is more common in women. A study of Nigerian patients with this symptom revealed 37.5% psychiatric morbidity compared with 12.5% in the control group (Saheeb and Otakpoor, 2005).

Similar associations between temporomandibular dysfunction and depression were found in a study of patients in Singapore (Yap *et al*, 2003). The results were compared with findings in American and Swedish studies and found to be similar. The vast majority of these subjects were women of child-bearing age.

It should be pointed out that in the case of jaw pain and dysfunction, this is not necessarily somatisation by the strict definition of the term, since in many cases an actual physical cause can be found in the form of arthritis of the jaw joints owing to teeth-grinding (bruxism) at night. The association with depressed women, however, is still valid.

Pelvic pain without apparent cause is also a finding among French women with high levels of psychological or neurotic problems (Dellenbach and Haerunger, 1996).

One must be careful to avoid assumptions about nationality and culture, social class, age and gender, without careful evaluation of the research evidence and appropriate comparisons. It is true that somatisation in general appears to be more common in Indian and Chinese subjects, women, and the elderly, when epidemiological data are analysed. However, in the studies mentioned above it is the researcher who has focused upon a specific symptom in a specific hospital department in a specific country. A common perception that the lower social classes display more somatisation than the more privileged, for instance, was found to be a myth, when challenged by research of 500 patients attending a pain clinic in the UK. In this study, pain, anxiety and depression scores were found to be distributed evenly throughout the social strata, as were the beneficial results of treatment (Larson and Marcer, 1984).

Also, somatisation is not confined to the realm of adults. Studies in Brazil and the US, each fairly large and focusing upon the ages 8 to 13 years, show an association between psychological illness and physical symptoms. The Brazil study showed anxiety associated with headache and teeth-grinding (Goyareb and Goyareb, 2002), while the study in the US showed how recurrent abdominal pain is strongly associated with both anxiety and depression in those children (Campo *et al*, 2004).

Many an astute parent has already observed how their child may introduce an emotional difficulty by saying, 'my tummy is hurting'.

Patterns of somatisation according to the mental health diagnosis

Anxiety disorders appear to produce a large variety of somatic symptoms. Headache, chest pain and abdominal pain are relatively common with anxiety, in addition to non-painful symptoms such as dizziness, shortness of breath and tremor. Research on pain has shown that the pain threshold is lowered in the anxious individual such that the pain is perceived more easily. But this only appears to occur when the anxiety is 'pain relevant', that is, when the subject is anxious about pain or a painful condition. When the focus of anxiety is some other issue, then the anxiety would appear to have a distracting effect on the subject's ability to feel pain (Lautenbacher and Krieg, 1994).

Panic disorder subjects appear to somatise at a higher rate than other forms of anxiety. One study of patients with panic disorder showed that 81% of them actually presented with a painful symptom. The most common was chest pain, followed by upper abdominal pain and then headache (along with dizziness and feeling faint) (Katon, 1984).

Depression and chronic pain are closely related. The state of depression renders the subject generally vulnerable to physical and emotional trauma, and this appears to include increased suffering of pain. Conversely, the chronic pain sufferer often is, or becomes, severely depressed. The association between depression and musculoskeletal pain, and jaw pain is mentioned above. Strangely, however, studies done to determine the pain threshold in depressed subjects seem to show that they are relatively *insensitive* to a deliberate pain stimulus, especially strong heat. The reason for this paradox is not fully understood. It is postulated that the particular pain symptoms in the depressive patient are related to false ideation or disturbances in perception. Also, the same factors that appear to produce a reduction in central alertness to a deliberate experimental painful stimulus may also, under usual circumstances, reduce central pain inhibitory mechanisms (Lautenbacher and Krieg, 1994).

In schizophrenia it has been thought that the pain threshold is higher than normal, and that this form of mental illness confers a kind of immunity or indifference to physical pain. This seems more connected with the 'attitude' of individual schizophrenics, the more withdrawn or chronic sufferer appearing indifferent to pain (Guieu *et al*, 1994). Another study suggests it may also be the use of antipsychotic medications which has a 'numbing' or pain-killing effect (Jakubaschk and Boker, 1991). Somatising pain patterns nevertheless occur in schizophrenics and are reported especially in the head, legs and back. These appear to be related to the specific delusional beliefs held by individual patients (Watson *et al*, 1981). The exact nature of pain perception in this group is thus unclear. Interestingly, when the well relatives of schizophrenics were tested, they showed a definite elevation of pain thresholds, suggesting that there may indeed be a genetic element (Hooley and Delgado, 2001).

There appears to be an association between chronic pain and borderline personality disorder. Chronic pain patients were tested by personality diagnostic questionnaires and semi-structured interviews for diagnosis of borderline personality disorder. Twenty-five per cent of the patients scored highly for this mental health problem, suggesting that chronic pain may be a manifestation of a self-regulatory disturbance amongst this group (Sansone *et al*, 2001). In a similar paradox to the depressive individuals, testing pain thresholds in subjects already diagnosed with personality disorders appears to show an increased threshold to pain. This was found to be especially so amongst those who practise self-mutilation, and it is thought that repeated and successive episodes of self-harm may have caused an adaptation process to render those subjects increasingly resistant to pain (Lautenbacher and Krieg, 1994).

Post-traumatic stress disorder subjects show a high incidence of chronic pain. Eighty per cent of Vietnam war veterans suffering from the disorder had somatising chronic pain related also to high pain disability scores (Beckham *et al*, 1997). Traumatised refugees in a refugee centre in Norway similarly showed a high incidence of chronic pain (65%). The pain did not appear to be related to the type, or degree, of the trauma originally suffered, but was associated with the presence of other diagnostic features of post-traumatic stress, anxiety and depression scores, and disability scores (Dahl *et al*, 2006). Holocaust survivors were also surveyed for chronic pain, and showed higher levels of pain, more sites of pain, and higher depression scores than the control group. Interestingly, unlike the Vietnam veterans, the Holocaust victims reported a higher than usual activity level, and did not consider themselves disabled (Yaari *et al*, 1999).

Sexual and physical abuse was found to be highly prevalent among a series of 167 consecutive chronic pain patients attending a pain clinic. Sixty-one per cent of these patients reported such abuse, related when carrying out semi-structured interviews. These patients were then compared with non-abused chronic pain sufferers, matching them for race, gender, pain type and time from onset of symptoms. The abused pain patients had a higher number of psychiatric diagnoses, greater distress levels, and a greater number of presentations to emergency departments prior to the start of treatment. Improvement after treatment, however, was the same in both groups, suggesting that the same techniques of treating chronic pain could be used for sufferers with different emotional histories (Bailey *et al*, 2003).

Issues in treatment, therapy and counselling

In dealing with this potentially complicated group of clients or patients, it is important, firstly, to be aware that somatisation is part of the mental health disorder. Failure to recognise this can hook the health professional into a difficult and unproductive personality conflict. A study showed that GPs find this group of individuals very difficult to deal with, miss the diagnosis of a mental health disorder, and consequently do not offer appropriate treatment, or treatment is poorly managed. After a brief training programme, however, those parameters greatly improved (Rosendal *et al*, 2005).

Having said this, the therapist must also be alert to the fact that real organic disease does occur even in the somatising subject. One does not want to encounter a 'cry wolf' situation in which a physical illness is missed because symptoms were assumed to be part of the client's emotional problem. The therapist or counsellor should not be reluctant or shy of seeking help from health professional colleagues, or encouraging the client to do so, should there be doubt.

The somatising individual is usually unaware that his/her pain and discomfort is part of a psychological problem and they may not take kindly to having this pointed out. Many a patient has attended the pain clinic with some resentment against their therapist or GP, declaring, 'He/she says it is all in my mind!' even though these were probably not the health professional's exact words (and even though, by definition, and as explained earlier, *all* pain perception *is* 'in the mind').

It is important to establish a rapport with the somatising client, and take their presentation of symptoms seriously. It is advisable not to become stuck in a 'which came first chicken or egg' way of thinking, that is, whether the pain has caused the depression or the depression has caused the pain. Regardless of the cause, the pain is real. A useful approach is to respect the client's belief that the pain is in the realm of the physical and apparently separate from the emotional. In the pain clinic, the physician, after establishing a good rapport, may suggest something like, 'It must be really distressing having so much pain. I am trying to help your pain as much as I can. Is anyone giving you support for the emotional stress?'. In the counselling room, the converse approach could be applied by the therapist: 'We are working together on some of your painful emotional issues. Is your doctor or nurse helping with the physical pain?'. Over the course of time, with both the physical and psychological aspects of the treatment exerting their influence, the client will hopefully come to integrate the two.

Even these suggestions can be misinterpreted if ill-timed or clumsily delivered. The individual must understand that he/she is not being passed off to someone else, but that additional treatment is being suggested. It is noteworthy that most pain programmes, under the auspices of the pain physician, include both mental health workers and physiotherapists in their team.

Another reason for separating treatment of the pain element from the emotional issues is illustrated by the fact that, for reasons not yet understood, these elements often respond to treatment at different rates. A study of depressed subjects with musculoskeletal pain treated with SSRI antidepressants showed that although both the depression and the pain improved in the first four weeks, the depression then continued to improve while the pain did not. This plateau of pain level lasted several months (Greco *et al*, 2004).

Much research has been carried out in order to establish what types of treatment are best suited to somatisation.

From the medication point of view, antidepressants would appear to help. The older tricyclic group (amitriptyline, imipramine) is well known to block pain impulses in the spinal cord, and this is given in doses much lower than that used for depression. The newer SSRI group is less effective for chronic pain. One group of patients, however, suffering from chronic fatigue syndrome, of which depression is a large component, appears to have improved considerably on the SSRI fluoxetine (Prozac) (Morris *et al*, 1999). This implies something different about the discomfort of chronic fatigue compared to other musculoskeletal disorders associated with depression.

The antipsychotic medication sulpiride has also been found to be useful. This was studied in a series of 669 somatisers, in combination with an exercise programme and CBT (Ferreri *et al*, 2000).

The importance of exercise is of note. It is well known in musculoskeletal and orthopaedic medicine that most musculoskeletal pain improves with exercise and worsens with lack of activity. It is also well established that depression lifts after exercise, probably because of the increase in norepinephrine (noradrenaline) and serotonin levels effected.

There exists, also, evidence for specific psychotherapies suited to the treatment of mental health problems associated with pain.

CBT would appear to be suitable for pain patients and has been much researched. One study evaluates this treatment in rehabilitation of adult chronic pain patients (Williams *et al*, 1993), while another assesses its use with children and adolescents (Garralda, 1999). Garralda (1999) looked at both populations, with positive outcomes. Pain therapists working in the team of a pain clinic or programme usually use this form of therapy. It may be that since pain is partly cognitive, some control is achieved by this method. In a pain programme, the psychotherapy will often include educational tutorials on the physiology of pain, as well as exercise advice and strategies for positive living and functioning along with the pain.

Anger management has been used to reduce pain sensitivity. However the form of anger management would appear to be critical, methods allowing anger expression being favoured over control or suppression (Burns *et al*, 2003).

Brief focal psychotherapy has been shown to help resolve chronic pain. This would appear to be especially suitable where deep unresolved issues of loss and mourning have not been addressed in the past. Exploration of these issues, and allowing their emotional content to be experienced by the client, can have a profound effect on resolution of the accompanying pain (Whale, 1992).

Finally, hypnosis has been considered for treatment of patients with pain. Most of us recall stage acts in which the hypnotised subject has a sharp object thrust through a skin fold without any apparent reaction or awareness. Whether it is possible or advisable to utilise this apparent method of pain control in mental ill-health with somatic symptoms are other matters. The theoretical basis has been studied using modern brain imaging and confirming those areas of the brain that modulate incoming pain impulses (the cingulate cortex referred to earlier). The important point here is that modulation of pain can be a consciously induced process (Kupers *et al*, 2005). Self-hypnosis has been taught to patients, usually by trained nursing staff, for both childbirth (Ketterhagen *et al*, 2002) and chronic pain sufferers (Buchser, 1999), with reported good effects. Upon closer scrutiny, this 'hypnosis' would appear to be another form of CBT and self-induced relaxation.

This chapter attempts to assist the therapist's understanding of the relationship between pain and mental health as well as explaining some of the possible mechanisms behind this link. When working with clients and patients, it can be useful to be aware of this association, in order that the therapy may go some way towards healing the classical 'mind–body split', a factor so often responsible for ill-health.

References

Bailey BE *et al* (2003) Lifetime physical and sexual abuse in chronic pain patients: psychosocial correlates and treatment outcomes. *Disability and Rehabilitation* 25:331–42.

Beckham JC *et al* (1997) Chronic posttraumatic stress disorder and chronic pain in Vietnam combat veterans. *Journal of Psychosomatic Research* 43:379–89.

Benzon HT *et al* (eds) (2005) *Essentials of Pain Medicine and Regional Anaethesia*. Philadelphia: Elsevier Churchill Livingstone.

Buchser E (1999) Hypnosis and self-hypnosis administered and taught by nurses for relief of chronic pain: a controlled clinical trial. *Forschende Komplementarmedizin* 6(Suppl. 1): 31–3.

Burns JW *et al* (2003) Emotional induction moderates effects of anger management style on acute pain sensitivity. *Pain* 106:109–18.

Campo JV *et al* (2004) Recurrent abdominal pain, anxiety and depression in primary care. *Pediatrics* 113:817–24.

Cheatle MD *et al* (1990) Chronic low back pain, depression and attributional style. *Clinical Journal of Pain* 6:114–17.

Creed F *et al* (eds) (1992) *Medical Symptoms not Explained by Organic Disease*. London: Gaskell.

Dahl S *et al* (2006) Chronic pain in traumatised refugees. *Tidsskrift for Den Norske Laegforening* 126:608–10.

Dellenbach P and Haerunger MT (1996) Chronic pelvic pain. Expression of a psychological problem. *Presse Medicale* 25:615–20.

Demiryoguran NS *et al* (2006) Anxiety disorder in patients with non-specific chest pain. *Emergency Medicine Journal* 23:99–102.

Ferreri M *et al* (2000) Sulpiride; a study of 669 patients with pain of psychological origin. *Encaphale* 26:58–66.

Garralda ME (1999) Practitioner review: assessment and management of somatization in childhood and adolescence: a practical perspective. *Journal of Child Psychology and Psychiatry and Allied Disciplines* 10:1159–67.

Goyareb MAM and Goyareb R (2002) Association between headache and anxiety disorders; indicators in a school sample from Ribeiroao Preto, Brazil. *Arqivos de Neuro-Psiquiatria* 60(3-B): 764–8.

Greco T *et al* (2004) The outcome of physical symptoms with treatment of depression. *Journal of General Internal Medicine* 19:813–18.

Green B (2003) Diagnosis and treatment of somatization. *Practitioner* 247:704–8.

Guieu R *et al* (1994) Objective evaluation of pain perception in patients with schizophrenia. *British Journal of Psychiatry* 164:253–5.

Hallstrom T and Posse M (1998) Depressive disorders among somatizing patients in primary health care. *Acta Psychiatrica Scandinavica* 98:187–92.

Hooley JM and Delgado ML (2001) Pain insensitivity in the relatives of schizophrenia patients. *Schizophrenia Research* 47:265–73.

Jakubaschk J and Boker W (1991) Disorders of pain perception in schizophrenia. *Schweitzer Archiv fur Neurologie und Psychiatrie* 142:55–76.

Kamaldeep B *et al* (2002) *Pocket Psychiatry*. Edinburgh and London: WB Saunders.

Katon W (1984) Panic disorder and somatization. Review of 55 cases. *American Journal of Medicine* 77:101–6.

Kendell RE (2001) The distinction between mental and physical illness. *British Journal of Psychiatry* 178:490–3.

Kendell RE and Zealley AK (eds) (1994) *Companion to Psychiatric Studies*. New York: Churchill Livingstone.

Ketterhagen D *et al* (2002) Self-hypnosis: alternative anesthesia for childbirth. *MCN, American Journal of Maternal Child Nursing* 27(6):335–40.

Kirkmayer LJ *et al* (1993) Somatisation and the recognition of depression and anxiety in primary care. *American Journal of Psychiatry* 150:734–41.

Kroenke K *et al* (1994) Physical symptoms in primary care: predictors of psychiatric disorders and functional impairment. *Archives of Family Medicine* 3:774–9.

Kupers R *et al* (2005) The cognitive modulation of pain: hypnosis and placebo-induced analgesia. *Progress in Brain Research* 150:251–69.

Larson AG and Marcer D (1984) The who and why of pain: analysis by social class. *British Medical Journal* 288:883–6.

Lautenbacher S and Krieg JC (1994) Pain perception in psychiatric disorders: a review of the literature. *Journal of Psychiatric Research* 28:109–22.

Morris RK *et al* (1999) Clinical and patient satisfaction outcomes of a new treatment for somatised mental disorder taught to general practitioners. *British Journal of General Practice* 49:236–67.

Raja SR and Dougherty PM (2005) Anatomy and physiology of somatosensory and pain processing. In: Benzon HT *et al* (eds) *Essentials of Pain Medicine and Regional Anesthesia*. Philadelphia: Elsevier Churchill Livingstone.

Rosendal M *et al* (2005) A randomised controlled trial of brief training in assessment of treatment of somatization. *Family Practice* 22:419–27.

Saheeb BD and Otakpor AN (2005) Co-morbid psychiatric disorders in Nigerian patients suffering temporomandibular joint pain and dysfunction. *Nigerian Journal of Clinical Practice* 8:23–8.

Sansone RA *et al* (2001) The prevalence of borderline personality among primary care patients with chronic pain. *General Hospital Psychiatry* 23:193–7.

Watson GD *et al* (1981) Relationship between pain and schizophrenia. *British Journal of Psychiatry* 138:33–6.

Williams AC *et al* (1993) Evaluation of a cognitive behavioural therapy programme for rehabilitation of patients with chronic pain. *British Journal of General Practice* 43:513–18.

Whale J (1992) The use of brief focal psychotherapy in treatment of chronic pain. *Psychoanalytical Psychotherapy* 6:61–72.

Yaari A *et al* (1999) Chronic pain in Holocaust survivors. *Journal of Pain and Symptom Management* 17:181–7.

Yap AU *et al* (2003) Prevalence of temporomandibular disorder subtypes, psychological distress and psychological dysfunction in Asian patients. *Journal of Orofacial Pain* 17:21–8.

Zwart JA *et al* (2003) Depression and anxiety disorders associated with headache frequency. *European Journal of Neurology* 10:147–52.

Chapter 9

Serious mental illness and dual diagnosis

Clare Gerada

Introduction

Many patients with serious enduring mental illness (SEMI) also have problems with drug and/or alcohol misuse. When the two are combined, the term dual diagnosis or co-morbidity is often used. Unfortunately the term is imprecise, as these patients seldom have just two problems. The combination of psychiatric and drug/alcohol problems means that individuals are at risk from a number of other problems, ranging from physical ill-heath, homelessness, unemployment, social exclusion and so on. Patients with both mental health problems and drug and alcohol problems are harder to retain in addiction, primary care and mental health services, and often fall through the gaps of service providers. The term 'multiple morbidity', suggested by Wright *et al* (2003), might more accurately describe the common predicament of patients who have more than one health problem. For the sake of brevity, the term dual diagnosis will be used in this chapter. These same patients will often be seen by counsellors, psychotherapists, psychologists and other healthcare workers in primary care.

What drugs are we talking about?

Levels of drug use are not static and change according to current vogue, price, availability and demographics of the population. Surveys show that over one in four of the UK population has used an illicit drug in their lifetime, with the highest rates found in 16–19 year olds (46%) and 20–29 year olds (41%). Use decreases in higher age groups to 12% at 50–59 years. Not surprisingly, cannabis is the most commonly used illicit drug and is likely to be taken frequently, with at least 9% of all users reporting daily use. About 100 000 people misuse heroin and an unknown but increasing number use other drugs such as ecstasy and amphetamines.

The number using crack-cocaine has been increasing since the 1990s and around 2–4% of the population use the drug on a regular basis. However, it is important to remember that most people who start using drugs stop taking them of their own volition, and most drug use is largely experimental and transient. It then would be highly probable that counsellors and psychotherapists are, have been or will be, working with individuals who have had experience with drug use, misuse and abuse. With this in mind, understanding of the terms and issues around drug use and co-morbidity become very relevant. Of course, it must be stated that not all individuals who have chemical or substance abuse issues have a SEMI or vice versa.

What is dependence/addiction?

The terms dependence and addiction are often used interchangeably, though strictly speaking the term dependence, when used alone, is a state of bodily adaptation to the presence of a certain psychoactive substance (tolerance) and manifests itself in physical disturbances or withdrawal symptoms when the substance is withdrawn. Not all drugs of misuse cause dependence, and not all those who use drugs are addicted. The term addiction or dependence syndrome refers to a specific psychological state in which the drug or other stimulus takes on an overriding importance in the person's life – when they do not have it they crave it. They plan their days around ensuring a regular supply of, or access to, the stimulus. A person can be addicted to activities other than drugs, such as gambling, playing computer games or indeed shopping; practitioners' listening and questioning in a sensitive manner may reveal more than initially met the eye, or ear.

Relationship between addiction and mental health problems

The relationship between those with addiction and serious mental health problems is complex, with possibilities for interrelationships (Crome, 1996) including:

- a primary psychiatric illness precipitating or leading to substance use
- substance use worsening or altering the course of a psychiatric illness, for example intoxication and/or substance dependence leading to psychological symptoms
- substance use and/or withdrawal leading to psychiatric symptoms or illnesses
- substances, particularly alcohol, cannabinoids, hallucinogens and stimulants (especially amphetamines and cocaine) can produce psychotic symptoms directly without mental illness.

Prevalence of dual diagnosis

The prevalence of dual diagnosis in the UK has increased over the last decade. This may be due to a number of factors, in particular:

- the general increase in substance use *per se* across the whole country means that patients with mental health problems are as likely (if not more so) to be caught up in the general increase in prevalence
- since the advent of care in the community, beginning in the late 1970s and continuing since then, patients with mental health problems are more exposed to drugs and hence more likely to use these substances than when incarcerated within long-stay asylums

- as certain drugs have become more prevalent in society, so their effects on those with genetic or other predispositions mean that these individuals are likely to develop serious mental health problems. This could be the reason for the increase in prevalence in psychotic illness in areas where cannabis use is particularly high, such as South East London.

Important epidemiological work has been conducted in the US. The American Epidemiological Catchments Area (ECA) study (Regier *et al*, 1990) surveyed over 20 000 people living in both community and psychiatric settings. Substance use problems were more prevalent among individuals with mental illness than among the general population, with mental illness, on average, doubling the chance of a co-existent substance use problem. The ECA study also reported the chances of lifetime substance use by diagnosis as follows:

- schizophrenia: 47%
- any bipolar disorder: 56%
- any affective disorder: 32%
- any anxiety disorder: 24%.

On this basis it appears that approximately half of those who experience serious mental illness will have a positive history of substance use (Mueser *et al*, 1995). A smaller-scale study of 171 people with psychosis in South London (Menezes *et al*, 1996) found that the one-year prevalence rate for any substance problem was 36.3%. Broken down further, 31.6% had alcohol problems, while 15.8% had drug problems. Young males were identified as being more likely to have substance use problems, and were found to have spent almost twice as long in hospital as those without such problems in the two-year period preceding the study. Significant mental health problems were also identified in opiate-dependent patients and amphetamine users in a South Wales drug dependence clinic (Barrowcliff *et al*, 1999).

The proportion of drug users with specific psychiatric conditions found in the UK National Treatment Outcome Research Study (NTORS) is shown in Table 9.1 (Marsden *et al*, 2000).

Table 9.1   The proportion of drug users with specific psychiatric conditions found in the NTORS study (Marsden *et al*, 2000)

Psychiatric disorder	Females (%)	Males (%)
Anxiety disorder	32	17
Depression	30	15
Paranoia	27	17
Psychotic	33	20

Using the General Practice Research Database in work commissioned by the Department of Health, Frischer *et al* (2000) looked at the prevalence of dual diagnosis in primary care in England and Wales from 1993–1998. The database recorded 1.4 million patient contacts with 230 practices. They checked for recorded individuals with both substance misuse and a psychiatric disorder and found that the rate for dual diagnosis increased by 62% during this period, with significant increases in schizophrenic disorder (128%), paranoia (144%), and psychotic disorder (147%). The authors also noted a regional variation, with a 300% increase in the Northern and Yorkshire district and a slow increase in London (Frischer *et al*, 2001). A study assessing the rates of dual diagnosis in five treatment settings in South London: primary care, specialist drug and alcohol community treatment services, mental health services, a forensic psychiatric service and primary care, using a screening tool, found high rates of dual diagnosis in all of these settings. Altogether 589 patients were screened, and just under half presented indications of dual diagnosis (*see* Table 9.2). This was the case for 83% of individuals from substance misuse services, more than one-third of whom, especially those with alcohol problems, also reported symptoms of psychosis. Around two-thirds of the substance misuse patients were identified as experiencing current depression and generalised anxiety. Though mild and moderate mental health problems were most prevalent in substance misuse services, SEMI was also found (Frischer *et al*, 2001).

Table 9.2 Percentage estimates of dual diagnosis in different treatment settings (Frischer *et al*, 2001)

Setting	Percentage with dual diagnosis
Community mental health patients	20
Psychiatric inpatients	43
Forensic patients	56
Substance misuse patients	83
Patients recruited through primary care	8

Brief summary of drugs of abuse

Benzodiazepines

Though not strictly speaking illicit (illegal) drugs, benzodiazepines are subject to abuse. Benzodiazepines are almost invariably used alongside heroin and cocaine, often in very large doses (for example, several 100 mg diazepam equivalents per day). Reasons for use are multifold and sometimes contradictory. They include to 'get high', to offset the stimulant effects of cocaine, or to prolong the hedonistic effects of heroin. This group of users should be differentiated from the long-term dependent iatrogenic users. This latter group tend to be elderly and use much lower doses initially prescribed as an anxiolytic or hypnotic.

A withdrawal syndrome can occur after only three weeks of continuous use, and it affects one-third of long-term users. The syndrome usually consists of increased anxiety and perceptual disturbances, especially heightened sensitivity to light and sound; occasionally there are fits, hallucinations, and confusion. Depending on the drug's half-life, symptoms start one to five days after the last dose, peak within 10 days, and subside after one to six weeks.

Opioids

Opioids (the term includes naturally occurring opiates such as heroin and opium, and synthetic opiates such as pethidine and methadone) produce an intense but transient feeling of pleasure. Withdrawal symptoms begin a few hours from the last dose, peak after two to three days, and subside after a week. Heroin is available in a powdered form, commonly mixed ('cut') with other substances such as chalk or lactose powder. It can be sniffed ('snorting'), eaten, smoked ('chasing the dragon'), injected subcutaneously ('skin popping'), or injected intravenously ('mainlining'). Tablets can be crushed and then injected.

Amphetamines

These cause generalised over-arousal with hyperactivity, tachycardia, dilated pupils, and fine tremor. These effects last about three to four hours, after which the user becomes tired, anxious, irritable, and restless. High doses and chronic use can produce psychosis with paranoid delusions, hallucinations, and over-activity. Physical dependence can occur, and termination of prolonged use may cause profound depression and lassitude. Amphetamines were widely prescribed in the 1960s: the most common current source is illegally produced amphetamine sulphate powder, which can be taken by mouth, by sniffing, or by intravenous injection. Metamphetamine ('ice', 'crystal' or 'glass') is chemically related to amphetamine but has more potent effects. It is associated with severe mental health problems.

Cocaine

Cocaine preparations can be eaten (coca leaves or paste), injected alone or with heroin ('speedballing'), sniffed ('snow'), or smoked (as 'crack'). Crack is cocaine in its base form and is smoked because of the speed and intensity of its psychoactive effects. The stimulant effect ('rush') is felt within seconds of smoking crack, peaks in one to five minutes, and wears off after about 15 minutes.

Smokable cocaine produces physical dependence with craving: the withdrawal state is characterised by depression and lethargy followed by increased craving, which can last up to three months. Overdose by any route can result in death from myocardial infarction, hyperthermia, or ventricular arrhythmias.

Cannabis

There are over 1000 different forms of cannabis, ranging from herbal varieties (marijuana, bush, grass, weed, draw), home-grown varieties ('skunk', 'northern lights') and resins ('soap bar', which accounts for roughly two-thirds of UK consumption and is typically combined with plastic, diesel to aid combustion and henna for colour). Cannabis is most commonly smoked, and it is in this form that it causes most harm to the lungs (lung cancer, bronchitis, asthma), and mental health problems (anxiety, paranoia, psychosis). There is some evidence that the potency of cannabis has increased in recent years. Around 5–10% of regular users develop dependence characterised by craving and withdrawal symptoms.

Patterns of drug and alcohol use

Research findings concerning the substances preferred by people with mental illness are equivocal. An early study (Schneier and Siris, 1987) reviewed patterns of drug use among people with schizophrenia. A propensity to use stimulants as a possible mechanism for alleviating negative symptoms was reported. However, the ECA study identified alcohol and cannabis to be the drugs most frequently used by individuals with schizophrenia (Frischer *et al*, 2000), and smaller UK studies have reported the same (McKeown and Liebling, 1995; Ryrie and McGowan, 1998).

Currently cannabis appears to be the illicit substance most commonly used by people with mental illness in the UK, mirroring the high use among those without mental health problems. Among the general population there is an increase in the availability of cocaine (Corkery, 2000; Boys *et al*, 1999) and a resurgence in heroin use in some cities (Eggington *et al*, 1998), and as any drug becomes more readily available we should expect increasing use to permeate many existing drug cultures including those with which psychiatric patients have contact.

Patients with schizophrenia have a three-fold greater risk of developing alcohol dependence compared to individuals without a mental illness (Crawford, 1996). The most common psychiatric disorder amongst injecting drug users is antisocial personality disorder (Drake and Noordsy, 1994).

Co-morbid mental health and substance use problems are especially prevalent in the homeless and rough sleepers and offenders, including prisoners. There are significant differences between men and women in their patterns of substance use and psychiatric co-morbidity (Department of Health, 2002). For example:

- women who use substances are significantly more likely than other women or men to have experienced sexual, physical and/or emotional abuse as children
- substance use lifestyles can impact on women's sexual health and establish a pattern of 're-victimisation'. For example, women are more likely to fund their habit through prostitution and hence are more likely to place themselves at risk of violence, assault and abuse
- women are more likely to present at mental health or primary care services for psychological difficulties rather than for any associated substance use problem
- women tend to access alcohol and drug services later than men and this may explain their more severe presentation
- women may have children, or want children, and this can deter them from contact with statutory services for fear that their children will be removed from them, meaning that they are likely to present later for care, at a time when their use has become more problematic.

Implications of substance use and mental health problems

The implications for people with mental health problems who also use drugs and/or alcohol can be serious, and it is important that the primary care practitioner is aware of them. Substance use among individuals with psychiatric disorders is associated with significantly poorer outcomes (Drake and Wallach, 1989; Carey *et al*, 1991; Kelly *et al*, 1995), including:

- worsening psychiatric symptoms
- increased rates of suicidal behaviour
- increased rates of violence (Smith *et al*, 1994)
- poor medication adherence
- increased risk of HIV infection
- higher service use
- higher rates of homelessness.

Both mental health problems and substance use are associated with higher rates of physical illness, including complications related to cigarette smoking, poor nutrition and infections, including tuberculosis. The primary care practitioner has an invaluable role in making sure that none of these problems are ignored.

Reasons for substance use

As we have seen people with mental illness are more likely to be using drugs and/or alcohol than people without. Several theories have been proposed to explain the high rates of substance use among people with schizophrenia (*see* Table 9.3; Siegfried, 1998).

Assessment of co-morbidity

Assessing a patient with dual diagnosis can be difficult; often the drug(s) used mask or add to psychiatric phenomenology. Ideally a period of abstinence is recommended before a full and accurate assessment of any underlying mental health problem can be made. The clinician should try and determine as fully as possible the pattern, severity and context of drug use and any causal relationship to the patient's mental health problems:

- *patterns of use*: the amounts of each substance used, frequency of use, length of time used, and by which route of administration
- *context of use*: personal and environmental factors that may be associated with an individual's drug use, including peer group attachments, positive and negative expectations of use and experiences of physical and/or psychological dependence. It is important also to ascertain protective factors, such as family support, appropriate housing and employment
- *severity of use*: patterns of use can give some indication of severity of dependence. This can be specified with instruments designed to gauge severity of alcohol use (Selzer, 1971), drug use (Raistrick *et al*, 1994; Marsden *et al*, 1998) and, more appropriately, substance use among individuals with serious mental illness (Drake *et al*, 1990)
- *assessment of risks*: including suicidal behaviour, aggressive or antisocial behaviour and blood-borne infections from sharing injecting equipment. An increased risk of accident might also be present. In addition the safety of prescribing a particular medication must be determined with regard to drug–drug interactions, but also how the medication is delivered or monitored.

Table 9.3   Theories about reasons for high rates of substance abuse among people with schizophrenia

Possible reasons for using drugs and/or alcohol	Comments
People with schizophrenia often use drugs and/or alcohol to self-medicate and to alleviate the side-effects of drugs.	Research evidence does not strongly support this view. For example, problematic alcohol use often precedes schizophrenia; specific drugs are not selected in relation to specific symptoms; importantly, various substances of use produce a range of different effects but generally exacerbate rather than relieve symptoms of schizophrenia (Chambers et al, 2001).
Underlying neuropathological abnormalities caused by schizophrenia facilitate the positive reinforcing effects of substance use and hence may predispose people to both conditions.	This may explain why people with schizophrenia prefer drugs such as cocaine and nicotine.
People with schizophrenia are especially vulnerable to the negative psychosocial effects of substance use, because schizophrenia impairs thinking and social judgement and induces poor impulse control.	This would explain why even when using small amounts of drugs and/or alcohol people with schizophrenia are prone to develop significant substance-related problems (Mueser et al, 1998).
People with antisocial personality disorder are at risk of developing substance use problems.	
The increased availability and acceptance of many substances in society mean that people with schizophrenia are more likely to come into contact with drugs and/or alcohol.	People with schizophrenia use substances for the same reasons as the general population, namely to enjoy the experience of intoxication, to escape from emotional distress and as a social activity (Lamb and Bachrach, 2001). Drug dealers can exploit people with an obvious vulnerability.

Treatment approaches

There is substantial evidence that treating substance use, especially opiate use, with the appropriate pharmacological and psychological interventions, helps improve outcome in a number of domains, including continued illicit use, criminal behaviour and social functioning. The National Treatment Outcome Research Study has estimated that every £1 spent on treatment saves £3 in criminal justice costs. The treatment of patients with dual diagnosis is of course complicated by the additional mental health problems, though there is no reason why the same treatment approaches as those used in those without a co-morbid problem cannot be used. However, practitioners need to have a realistic and long-term view of treatment and it is important that they are aware of the different approaches that may be necessary during different stages of treatment.

The following stages of treatment have been described:

* engagement
* motivation for change
* active treatment
* relapse prevention.

Which do you treat first?

Management should of course involve the two problematic elements, namely treating the substance of use and treating any co-existing mental health problem. Three approaches are currently used for delivering services to patients, and the choice of course depends on local circumstances. The GPwSI may have an important role in determining which service is commissioned. Whatever model is used, a most important aspect of any service is the ability to be flexible and to offer services that meet the needs of that individual patient, at the time they present.

A Cochrane review (Ley *et al*, 2000) of different interventions found little evidence to support the effectiveness of any particular treatment, or to recommend one approach over any other. However the research does suggest a growing agreement that integrated mental health and substance use services offer a more tolerant, non-confrontational approach for patients and are probably the best and most appropriate way forward for these patients. Champney-Smith (2002) makes the point that whatever the model of service provided, there are a number of steps that should be considered in order to maximise the effectiveness of treatment:

* comprehensive assessments of both mental health and substance use problems
* training for mental health workers in the recognition and management of substance use problems
* training for substance use workers in the recognition and management of mental health problems
* services that are non-judgemental, flexible and take account of the principles of harm minimisation
* assertive outreach with appropriate case loads

- clear understanding of roles and responsibilities
- good liaison between agencies, clearly identifying who has the lead
- development of care pathways.

Evaluation of new services using a range of outcome measures

Whatever model of care is used to deliver services, close communication and effective shared care between all those involved are important. Practitioners with special clinical interest may have a role in supporting patients with dual diagnosis, helping them move across the many interfaces of care, but all primary care practitioners will play an important role.

Pharmacological interventions

The pharmacological interventions for patients with dual diagnosis are broadly similar to those for other patients with addiction problems. The mainstay of treatment of opiate dependence is maintenance substitute medication, either with methadone mixture or with buprenorphine. Details of treatment are beyond the scope of this chapter and the reader is advised to consult fuller texts for more detailed pharmacological treatments.

Psychological interventions

Counselling has been used widely in helping people to deal with their drug or alcohol misuse, or more specifically, to help people to deal with negative emotions and behaviours that become cues to use drugs or alcohol. Cognitive-behavioural therapy (CBT) is useful in demonstrating to the patient self-destructive, sabotaging behaviours that he may be unaware of. Less well known but very useful is cognitive analytic therapy which aims to create with patients narrative and diagrammatic re-formulations of their difficulties, and has the added benefit of being time limited and hence inexpensive.

Cue exposure and coping skills training or variations on that theme form the basis of the generic strategy known as 'relapse prevention'. Group therapy may be nothing more than self-help groups of patients discussing common problems and common strategies. Shared experiences and treatment can be very powerful: they allow greater insights into a person's behaviour by using the perspectives of others in the group who may have identified similar problems in themselves. Groups act as a 'resonance chamber', within which an individual will have his reactions and behaviours amplified for all to see. Groups confer the additional benefit of increasing self-efficacy by using the observations of the patients themselves to be therapeutic.

'Twelve step' or 'Minnesota Method' groups have been an extraordinary phenomenon since their inception in the 1940s. The original groups set themselves up with no professional input to address their alcohol dependency and became known as 'Alcoholics Anonymous' (AA). As the years have passed, the same philosophy has been extended to all addictive drugs (Narcotics Anonymous), specific drugs such as cocaine (CA), and also sex (SA), gambling (GA) and other behaviours that are banded together as 'addictions'. AA groups are available in most cities in the world and many smaller country areas as well. They remain 'anonymous', in as much as they are open only to those who admit to their dependency and ask for help – there is no trained or professional input, and each group will behave in slightly different ways, reflecting the different personalities within it.

Contrary to widely held belief, they are not faith based as such, in that you do not have to hold a religious belief, but 'The Steps' (toward recovery) become a sort of faith in themselves – that if you admit to the group your powerlessness over your addiction and ask for help, and if you keep to the programme, you will achieve sustained abstinence. The language employed can be arcane and off-putting to some, but there are a number of studies showing a close correlation between 'twelve step' meeting attendances, and duration of abstinence.

What can the primary care professional do?

It is the author's belief that the more complex the individual, the more they need the services of well-organised primary care. Of course GPs should not act in isolation, and a multiprofessional approach to care optimises treatment opportunities. However, with many carers involved in treating the different needs of the patient it is easy for them to fall through service gaps and for the age-old problem of poor communication between services to undermine care. Key working is important, and it is not proposed that the GP or primary care nurse takes over this role. However, the stability and familiarity of the GP and their team with the complete patient record mean that it seems natural that the GP can and should provide the focal point for liaison between agencies in these complex cases. Box 9.1 summarises what primary care can offer to patients with dual diagnosis.

Box 9.1 What can primary care offer to patients with dual diagnosis?

- Co-ordination of care between different service providers
- Continuity of care
- Care of complex needs
- Crisis intervention
- Provision of general medical services
- Care to the family
- Medication review
- Advocacy

Conclusion

Patients with drug misuse problems and co-existing mental health problems have complex needs. These needs can be met by existing primary care services working in partnership with other health and social care services. Treatment works and it is important that these patients are given every opportunity to access help.

References

Barrowcliff A, Champney-Smith J and McBride A (1999) The opiate treatment index (OTI). Treatment assessment with Welsh samples of opiate prescribed or amphetamine prescribed clients. *Journal of Substance Use* 4:98–103.

Boys A, Marsden J and Griffiths P (1999) Reading between the lines: is cocaine becoming the stimulant of choice for urban youth? *Druglink* 14:20–3.

Carey M, Carey K and Meisler A (1991) Psychiatric symptoms in mentally ill chemical abusers. *Journal of Nervous and Mental Disease* 179:136–8.

Chambers A, Krystal JH and Self DW (2001) A neurobiological basis for substance abuse comorbidity in schizophrenia. *Biological Psychiatry* 50:71–83.

Champney- Smith J (2002) Dual diagnosis. In: Petersen T and McBride A (eds) *Working with Substance Users: a guide to theory and practice*. London: Routledge, pp. 267–74.

Corkery J (2000) *Drug Seizure and Offender Statistics, United Kingdom 1998: Home Office statistical bulletin 3/00*. London: Home Office Research Development and Statistics Directorate.

Crawford V (1996) Comorbidity of substance use and psychiatric disorders. *Current Opinion in Psychiatry* 9:231–4.

Crome I (1996) *Psychiatric Disorder and Psychoactive Substance use Disorder: Towards improved service provision*. London: Centre for Research into Drugs and Health Behaviour.

Department of Health (2002) *Mental Health Policy Implementation Guide: dual diagnosis good practice guide*. London: HMSO.

Drake R and Noordsy D (1994) Case management for people with co-existing severe mental disorder and substance abuse disorder. *Psychiatric Annals* 24:427–31.

Drake R, Osher F, Noordsy D et al (1990) Diagnosis of alcohol use disorders in schizophrenia. *Schizophrenia Bulletin* 16:57–67.

Drake R and Wallach M (1989) Substance abuse among the chronic mentally ill. *Hospital and Community Psychiatry* 40:1041–6.

Eggington R, Parker H and Bury C (1998) Heroin still screws you up: responding to new heroin outbreaks. *Druglink* 13:17–20.

Frischer M, Hickman M, Kraus L et al (2001) A comparison of different methods for estimating the prevalence of problematic drug misuse in Great Britain. *Addiction* 96: 1465–76.

Kelly J, Heckman T, Helfrich S et al (1995) HIV risk factors and behaviours among men in a Milwaukee homeless shelter. *American Journal of Public Health* 85:465–8.

Lamb HR and Bachrach L (2001) Some perspectives on deinstitutionalization. *Psychiatric Services* 52:1039–45.

Ley A, Jeffrey DP, McLaren S and Siegfried N (2000) Treatment programmes for people with both severe mental illness and substance use (Cochrane Review), *The Cochrane Library Issue 1*. Oxford: Update Software.

Marsden J, Gossop M and Stewart D (1998) The Maudsley Addiction Profile (MAP): a brief instrument for assessing treatment outcomes. *Addiction* 93:1857–68.

Marsden J, Gossop M, Stewart D et al (2000) Psychiatric symptoms among clients seeking treatment for drug dependence: intake data from the National Treatment Outcome Research Study. *British Journal of Psychiatry* 176:285–9.

McKeown M and Liebling H (1995) Staff perceptions of illicit drug use within a special hospital. *Journal of Psychiatric and Mental Health Nursing* 2:343–50.

Menezes P, Johnson S, Thornicroft G et al (1996) Drug and alcohol problems among individuals with severe mental illnesses in South London. *British Journal of Psychiatry* 168:612–19.

Mueser K, Bennett M and Kushner M (1995) Epidemiology of substance use disorders among persons with chronic mental illness. In: Lehman A and Dixon L (eds) *Double Jeopardy: chronic mental illness and substance use disorders.* Chur, Switzerland: Harwood Academic, pp. 9–25.

Mueser KT, Drake RE and Wallach MA (1998) Dual diagnosis: a review of etiological theories. *Addictive Behaviours* 23:717–34.

Raistrick D, Bradshaw J, Tober G *et al* (1994) Development of the Leeds Dependence Questionnaire (LDQ): a questionnaire to measure alcohol and opiate dependence in the context of a treatment evaluation package. *Addiction* 89:563–72.

Regier D, Farmer M, Rae D *et al* (1990) Comorbidity of mental disorders with alcohol and other drug use. *Journal of the American Medical Association* 264:2511–18.

Ryrie I and McGowan J (1998) Staff perceptions of substance use among acute psychiatric in-patients. *Journal of Psychiatric and Mental Health Nursing* 5:137–42.

Schneier F and Siris S (1987) A review of psychoactive substance use and abuse in schizophrenia: patterns of drug choice. *Journal of Nervous and Mental Disease* 175:641–52.

Selzer M (1971) The Michigan Alcoholism Screening Test: the quest for a new diagnostic instrument. *American Journal of Psychiatry* 127:1653–8.

Siegfried N (1998) A review of comorbidity: major mental illness and problematic substance use. *Australian and New Zealand Journal of Psychiatry* 32:707–17.

Smith J, Frazer S and Boer H (1994) Dangerous dual diagnosis patients. *Hospital and Community Psychiatry* 45:280–1.

Wright N, Smeeth L and Heath I (2003) Moving beyond single and dual diagnosis in general practice. *British Medical Journal* 326:512–14.

Chapter 10

Critical appraisal: how to find the evidence on severe and enduring mental illness

Joan Curzio

Introduction

Many of the authors in this book make reference to a variety of research reports that provide the 'evidence' for counselling, psychotherapy or mental health practice. In response, this chapter is about grappling with what research evidence there is that supports the identification and management of individuals with diagnoses that fall within the scope of severe and enduring mental illness (SEMI). Much of the information in this chapter will help individuals develop the critical appraisal skills necessary in writing essays, doing a degree, conducting research, or simply looking for the evidence. It has become increasingly important, particularly in the field of counselling, to generate research to inform primary and secondary care and further this profession.

With the advent of the evidence-based practice movement within healthcare (Evidence-Based Medicine Working Group, 1992; Rosenberg and Donald, 1995) and the ready availability of a wide range of systematic reviews of research, it is generally accepted that such evidence will be used. In fact, the NHS clinical governance policy within the UK demands that wherever possible, research be used to demonstrate the clinical effectiveness of the care being offered (Department of Health, 1999). This is becoming a 'way of life' in healthcare, and will affect counselling, as well as other areas of psychological and mental health.

Unfortunately, most of the work that has been done to synthesise mental healthcare research results has focused on quantitative studies of drug treatments. A recent survey of the Cochrane database of systematic reviews (www.cochrane. org/) to look for reviews in the care of schizophrenia found 78 reviews, the vast majority dealing with drug treatment and only 16 dealing with non-pharmacological interventions and other aspects of care. While there is a preponderance of pharmacologically focused systematic reviews and studies, there is a growing evidence base exploring a variety of issues around the non-drug treatment of people with one or more of the diagnoses within SEMI.

What follows is an attempt to summarise a range of techniques that counsellors and others can use to identify, find, filter, and critique the quantitative and qualitative research for practice. However, it is outside the scope of this chapter to describe how each individual clinician could incorporate that evidence into their practice.

Definitions

Critical appraisal can be defined as the evaluation of relevant research evidence using an organised systematic approach to determine its usefulness for clinical practice.

Muir Gray (1996) defines *evidence-based practice* as that which uses research evidence in conjunction with the values of both patients and healthcare professionals and the resources available to provide that care. This is a useful definition, as it broadens out the definition beyond the slavish implementation of research results to include interpretation and contextualisation of those results.

Identifying the evidence

The first thing that needs to be done is to find the evidence. Today this is far simpler than in the past. There is no longer any need to trawl through individual volumes of *Index Medicus* that contained vast lists of authors, titles of papers and journal details broadly indexed by topic. Now this information, plus much more (*see* Box 10.1) is recorded in a range of bibliographic databases and search engines that can be readily searched electronically, a number of which (*see* Table 10.1) are updated regularly. Even though many contain references to the same journals and articles, if a thorough search is needed, more than one database should be explored.

Box 10.1   General content of a bibliographic database entry for a journal article

- Author or authors
- Title
- Year of publication
- Journal title
- Volume number
- Issue number
- Page numbers
- Abstract
- Keywords
- Language written in

Table 10.1   Bibliographic databases and searching sites

Name of database	Description of focus
ASSIA	Sociological information
CINAHL	Nursing and allied health literature
Cochrane databases	Systematic reviews
MEDLINE, PubMed	General medical information
PsychInfo	Psychological information
SCOPUS	Scientific, technical and medical (includes all of MEDLINE and other basic science information)
Zetoc	British Library's current journals and conference proceedings from 1993
GOOGLE Scholar (http://scholar.google.com/)	Web-based search engine for scholarly literature

Once one has found a relevant article, additional relevant material may be found by reading through the reference list of the article. This is referred to as secondary searching. Authors who have published one paper on a topic may well have written others, so it can be worthwhile to do an author search on each of the authors of a paper in each of the bibliographic databases being searched. There may also be specific journals that publish papers in the same or similar areas of interest (*see* Box 10.2). The table of contents of these can be reviewed either during a visit to a local library that has that journal or online on the journal or publisher's website.

Box 10.2   A sample of journals that regularly publish research articles on diagnoses that fall within SEMIs

- *Acta Psychiatrica Scandinavia*
- *Archives of General Psychiatry*
- *British Journal of Psychiatry*
- *Current Opinion in Psychiatry*
- *Drugs and Alcohol Dependence*
- *International Journal of Mental Health Nursing*
- *International Journal of Psycho-Analysis*
- *International Journal of Social Psychiatry*
- *Journal of the American Academy of Child Psychiatry*
- *Primary Care Psychiatry*
- *Psychiatry*
- *Psychological Medicine*
- *Schizophrenia Bulletin*
- *The Psychologist*

Once searching commences, it generally becomes clear who are the 'experts' researching and publishing on the topic. It is recommended, for those searching for research reports for systematic reviews, that these experts be contacted and asked if they have or know of any reports not already obtained by the searcher.

In addition to the above, individual counsellors, psychotherapists and other similar professionals who wish to keep up to date with the current research can do so in several ways. This can easily be done by subscribing to and reading one or more of the journals listed in Box 10.2 or similar publications. Scanning content tables on journal or publisher websites can be useful too, while joining a journal club can also be a way of finding and appraising literature (more on this later).

With the advent of the worldwide web and search engines such as Google and Yahoo, it is quite easy to find vast quantities of information on any topic. However, there is yet to be a 'vetting' system for information posted online. The searcher needs to take care and consider the veracity of any and all information obtained in this way. The evidence for clinical practice should come from peer-reviewed publications, i.e. those articles that have been critiqued by two 'peers' in that clinical/research area and approved by them for publication. Fortunately there are a growing number of websites that either access or hold peer-reviewed publications (*see* Table 10.2).

Table 10.2 Websites for accessing research reports

Website address	Description
www.nelh.nhs.uk/	National library for health programme website funded by the UK Department of Health
www.biomedcentral.com	E-journals that are freely accessible
www.freemedicaljournals.com	Gateway to accessing free a number of medical and nursing journals, some only after a specific period of time, such as *New England Journal of Medicine* after 6 months

In addition, there are evidence-based newsletters, which can be useful sources. The most famous of these is Bandolier (www.jr2.ox.ac.uk/bandolier/). Its website is a bastion of clearly written critique of available evidence in primary care, and a number of their articles relate to mental health topics.

Search techniques

Every bibliographic database has its own 'interface', so that each has its own look and feel. They all have a box where terms are entered with a 'Search' or 'Find' button that initiates the search. Searches to identify research publications for systematic reviews can be quite complex (*see* the latest edition of the Cochrane Handbook available on their website: www.cochrane.org/). However, much can be found using a few simple techniques. Start by using terms you would use to identify the topic. For example, if a clinician wished to find the treatments and their outcomes for manic depression, the words: 'manic depression' can be entered. If a large number of articles are identified, this search can be refined by combining the number of this search with the term: 'treatment' in the following manner:

'1 and treatment'

There are other refinements, for example, the CINAHL database has option buttons below their search box that can be checked. These include selecting for research, English language, and full text available. On other databases these refinements can be added to the search as described above. Searching based on methodological approaches can also be helpful. Work looking at retrieving relevant mental health intervention studies from MEDLINE found that combining indexing terms identifying methodologies with descriptive words yielded far fewer irrelevant publications (Wilczynski and Haynes, 2006).

Work has also progressed on the development of what are referred to as filters or hedges (Haynes *et al*, 1994) and other tools (Dong *et al*, 2004; Fontelo *et al*, 2005) that allow clinicians and other searchers to access relevant publications more easily. Many of these do take some effort to master, but can help focus searches. While some have shown good results (Haynes *et al*, 1994; Berg *et al*, 2005), a systematic evaluation has identified limitations as not all filters have found substantial proportions of relevant papers (Jenkins, 2004).

Many libraries offer sessions covering how to access bibliographic databases and the basic search techniques. In addition, librarians are usually happy to help if trouble is encountered.

Finding the evidence

Scan the list of titles found by each search and read the abstracts of the papers that appear relevant, ticking the ones of interest. Next, print out or save them using the option that gives the abstract as well as the basic reference details for those selected.

Once articles of interest are identified, these need to be found. Some of the bibliographic databases have full-text links which allow for immediate access to an electronic copy of the article. This can then be either printed or saved electronically for further study. A number of journals have websites, and for many readers can access individual articles, for a price. However, there is also a website where copies of a range of international medical journals can be found free of charge (www.freemedicaljournals.com). Plus, there is a growing movement of open access journals that are peer reviewed and available to anyone via the internet. One such group of journals can be found at BioMed Central (www.biomedcentral.com). Finally, many NHS trusts have access to NHSNet (www.nhsia.nhs.uk/nhsnet), which requires a password, but provides links to a range of bibliographic databases, and electronic access to full-text journal articles.

Most NHS organisations either have their own library or have access to a local healthcare library. Frequently they operate informal interlibrary exchange schemes that health librarians support by photocopying articles from journals in their library in exchange for copies of articles from journals held by other health libraries locally. In addition, libraries can access the interlibrary loan scheme from the British Library, although this option does incur charges.

Critiquing the evidence

A general approach

All research, whether in counselling, medicine or technology, regardless of the methodology or methodological approach used (*see* Table 10.3) has the same process, and therefore reports of any type of research will generally have a common structure:

- an introduction that gives background to the study
- an aim with or without objectives
- a methods section of how the study was undertaken and analysed
- a description of the subjects or population studied
- a description of the data or information collected
- a summary of the results
- a discussion of the results, frequently putting them into context with previously published research
- conclusions.

Table 10.3 Broad research methodologies

Methodology	Description
Quantitative	Objective, systematic process to collect numerical information from which generalisable conclusions are drawn
Qualitative	Subjective, systematic approach that usually explores people's perceptions, understandings and interpretations of life experiences to give them meaning
Action research	A step-by-step exploratory approach that is an iterative process using either qualitative or quantitative techniques where little is known. Each step informs the next

When critiquing any research article, the reader needs to consider whether or not the introduction and background sections not only 'set the scene' but justify conducting the study. Thus, the need for the study should be made apparent. This is done through citing previous research in this area, including, where appropriate, identifying the strengths and weaknesses in that research. When looking at the references, there should be a spread of publication dates. If all research cited is more than a few years old, then recent work may have been overlooked. Alternatively, if only work published in the last two years is cited, then important previous work may have been omitted.

The aim or question being addressed in the study needs to be clearly stated and do-able. Many articles have a specific section entitled: 'Aims' or 'Aims and objectives', but at times, these may not be easy to identify. When the latter is the case, look to the last line of the introduction and/or background section, where it may be stated. Occasionally it can be found as the first line of the discussion section.

The reader needs to consider whether or not the method used is capable of answering the aim of the study with the identified population in the environment used. In addition, ask: was the time taken adequate to answer the aim with the identified population in the environment used?

It is just as important, in counselling research, as it is in any other research to consider whether or not the subjects were an appropriate group with which to do the study. Were there a sufficient number recruited? If there is a control or comparison group, are the subjects in each from the same population? Finally, did subjects drop out? If so, how many subjects withdrew and for what reason?

The data or information collected need to be capable of answering the aims and objectives of the study. If some data were not collected or are missing for any reason, if clients did not attend for example, how much data were not collected and what steps the researchers have taken to cope with this, all should be described by the authors.

Data analysis needs to be appropriate to the data and also has to be capable of answering the aim and objectives. Small studies with a small amount of quantitative data lend themselves to simple analysis, although if percentages are reported, the authors should include the numbers from which they were calculated. Readers should be concerned if complex analysis has been done with a very small dataset, as most complex statistical analysis requires reasonably sized groups for comparison. If the reader is in doubt, someone with greater statistical knowledge can be consulted.

The discussion section of any paper should put the results in context with other work done in the area. This should include some critique of both the published work and the current study. There should be an acknowledgement of the limitations of the study. No one study can sort out or explore every issue or concern in the area being researched.

Finally, the conclusions should be drawn from the question under study and the results of the analysis. Some authors are tempted to overstate their results, while others lend more trustworthiness to their conclusions when presented cautiously:

- 'These results indicate . . .'
- 'These results add to the growing body of knowledge . . .'.

Specific issues to consider when reading a quantitative study

In addition to the guidance given above, there are a number of issues one needs to consider when reading a quantitative study, particularly if it is a randomised controlled trial (RCT). Although most counselling and psychotherapy research may not lend itself to this kind of approach, knowledge of the different studies can be useful when seeking to understand different kinds of studies. An RCT is a comparison study, generally of an intervention, where subjects from the same population have been selected to join one of the groups under study via random allocation. Alternating group allocation is not randomisation. There is a range of computer programmes and random number tables that can support randomisation activities. This is the sort of information that should be provided to readers regarding which randomisation techniques have been used.

The size of the population in a quantitative study is important; larger groups are more likely to give more robust answers to questions. However, since resources to undertake research are frequently limited, researchers use what is called a power calculation to determine the size of group they need to recruit. Thus, if researchers state that their study has a 95% power, that means that if that study was done with that number of subjects 100 times, then 95 times they would get the same answer they got this time.

'Blinding' is where the subjects are not informed which group they have been allocated to, while 'double-blinding' means that the researchers conducting the study also don't know the group to which the subjects have been allocated. This is considered a means of reducing bias within a study. An additional method to reduce bias in an intervention study is to have a different person carry out the evaluation of the outcomes.

The measurement tools used in any quantitative study should be shown to accurately measure the outcome they are said to be measuring. This is called reporting the validity (does it measure what it is purporting to measure?) and the reliability (does it do so repeatedly?) of outcome measures.

Some quantitative research requires complex statistical tests to enable an answer to the question(s) posed. These can be quite daunting for the clinical reader who may only be able to note whether or not the P value presented is less than 0.05, indicating statistical significance. The P value indicates the likelihood or probability of the difference found between the groups under study occurring by chance. If unsure, there may be a local researcher with statistical knowledge who is willing to discuss the analysis and its interpretation.

Finally, the overall quality of published RCT papers has improved in the last 10 years. This is due in large part to the editors of international medical journals agreeing a standard for their publication entitled the CONSORT statement (Begg *et al*, 1996).

Limitations of quantitative research within counselling and mental health services

Quantitative studies are predicated upon there being clearly defined diagnoses, large enough populations in which to conduct studies and standardised measurable clinical outcomes. However, the fact that this will frequently not be the case within the care of mentally ill individuals has been acknowledged (Barnes *et al*, 1999).

Specific issues to consider when reading a quantitative systematic review

A systematic review attempts to identify, critique and synthesise all published and unpublished research that has been done to answer a question. In its simplest form, it will be descriptive. However, quantitative studies that utilise the same outcome measure provide scope for the summing of results across a number of similar studies (meta-analysis). The results of a meta-analysis are considered the most powerful to inform healthcare decisions, as they establish whether results are consistent, and can be applied across groups, settings and different doses (Grimshaw *et al*, 2003).

The Cochrane Collaboration was established to facilitate the development and use of systematic reviews. Their website holds databases of completed reviews, protocols, other relevant information and access to their methodologies (www.cochrane.org/). Due to financial constraints, the full database has been taken over by the Wiley publishing company, and unless one is accessing it via an organisation with a subscription, only titles and abstracts are available. However, as outlined above, most healthcare professionals within the NHS have access through the NHSnet gateway (www.nelh.nhs.uk/cochrane.asp). NHS counsellors may need to request help to access it through their NHS place of work. Generally universities with health faculties will have subscriptions as well.

To minimise bias and random errors within a systematic review, a number of steps need to be taken and these are identified in detail in the *Cochrane Handbook* (www.cochrane.org/). Since knowing what these steps are can help a reader critique a review, they are broadly summarised here.

The authors of a systematic review need to clearly state the question the review is attempting to answer, the search terms used and where they searched (including checking reference lists of relevant articles, table of contents of relevant journals, identifying 'grey literature' and contacting experts for unpublished reports). The criteria used to include and exclude studies from the review, methods used to summarise or pool results and the conclusions drawn need to be identified. The team of reviewers needs to include a range of clinical and research experts, including statistical expertise if a meta-analysis is being undertaken.

When a meta-analysis is undertaken as part of the systematic review, the report needs to include an assessment of whether or not the variability within the results from each study being pooled is roughly similar (homogeneous) or is different (heterogeneous). If heterogeneity has been detected, the results from these studies should not be pooled and need to be reported separately. Further discussion of this point and other finer points of critically appraising systematic reviews with and without meta-analysis can be found in Greenhalgh (1997).

Specific issues to consider when reading a qualitative study

Qualitative research explores individuals' experience, perceptions, meanings and understanding and provides opportunities for the generation of hypotheses and insights into meaning. The differences from quantitative research lie within its subjectivity, inductive processes and depth of exploration seeking understanding, not overt generalisability.

Although there is a range of qualitative methodological approaches (*see* Table 10.4), they can all use the same techniques: interviews, focus groups, diaries, observation, etc. The differences are in the underlying philosophical approach used that then dictates who should be recruited and how data are collected (for example: the form the interview questions take), analysed and interpreted. The position of the researcher is paramount. This should be clearly stated with the author's perspective identified and the potential for any bias or influence noted. Therefore, taking in the above considerations, the reader should look at the question being posed, the method or methodologies used, the subjects recruited,

Table 10.4 Examples of qualitative research approaches

Approach	Brief description	Further information/proponents
Grounded theory	Develops theory 'grounded' in subjects' interaction in a social scene	Glaser and Strauss were the first proponents (summarised briefly in Glaser, 2002)
Phenomenology	Attempts to understand the whole human through the 'lived experience' of subjects	Husserl, Heidegger and Gadamer (summary of each of their perspectives can be found in Laverty, 2003)
Ethnography	Studies members of a culture, explores the impact of culture on human behaviour	Agar, 1997
Content analysis	Sits within the broad qualitative or naturalistic paradigm (approach). Interprets the meaning of the content of textual data	Hsieh and Shannon, 2005
Thematic analysis	Sits within the broad qualitative or naturalistic paradigm (approach)	Miles and Huberman, 1994; Boyatzis, 1998

the data obtained and how those data were analysed, interpreted and reported. Differences in a counsellor's theoretical orientation for example, such as person-centred or psychodynamic, may affect the position they take in approaching their topic, as well as how they explain their results.

Direct quotes from the research participants are usually presented; this allows the reader to check for themselves the linkage between what the subjects have said and the interpretation put upon it by the researchers. Further details of how to critically appraise qualitative research can be found in Greenhalgh (1997); Horsburgh (2002); and a series of three articles published in the *British Medical Journal* (Mays and Pope, 2000; Pope *et al*, 2000; Meyer, 2000).

Specific issues to consider when reading qualitative or other types of systematic review

As systematic review techniques were specifically designed around the analysis of quantitative studies (*see* previous discussion), it has taken time for the role of qualitative research to emerge. Techniques for conducting qualitative systematic reviews have been described (Jones, 2004) along with the use of 'meta-synthesis' (Pawson, 2002), while another set of authors has suggested that using qualitative techniques to integrate results from studies using a range of qualitative method-ologies can be utilised to conduct what they refer to as an 'integrative review' (Whittemore and Knafl, 2005). There has yet to be a systematic approach pro-posed for the critical appraisal of the outputs of these techniques.

However, as seen from the previous discussion, a basic approach can be taken. The reader can look to:

- the question being posed
- the techniques used to discover the research to be included
- inclusion and exclusion criteria used
- ways the results were analysed and presented.

Again, the role the researchers had in the process needs to have been clearly identified.

Specific issues to consider when reading a single case study report

Generally single case studies are not considered as evidence for evidence-based practice. Stickley and Phillips (2005) and Welsh and Lyons (2001) all argue that, while single case studies are not evidence for generalisability, they do offer analytical generalisability, particularly in the mental health nursing care arena.

As with the other critical approaches described above, the reader should be systematic when reading a case study.

Developing critical appraisal skills

Critical appraisal skills are best developed through discussing papers with other people who are also interested in the subject of the paper under discussion. Reading a chapter like this one, an article (Fowkes and Fulton, 1991) or book

(Greenhalgh, 1997) covering critical appraisal is a good way to get started. Most trust research and development departments run critical appraisal workshops or can refer healthcare professionals to those available locally.

Many people have found participation in a journal club helpful. These are regular meetings, formal or informal, where a group of interested healthcare professionals gather to discuss a paper or several papers. Journal clubs can be organised in several ways, including being organised so that one member reads the paper quite closely in order to lead the discussion, while in other clubs, everyone reads the paper and there is a general discussion. Journal clubs have been found to be a helpful learning tool when introducing evidence-based practice (Cramer and Mahoney, 2001) and the usefulness in psychiatry has also been highlighted (Swift, 2004). For details on how to run one please see the Swift (2004) paper in the reference list. In addition, during the preparation of this chapter, a number of papers looking at a variety of aspects of SEMIs were identified (*see* Box 10.3).

Such skills could assist counsellors and psychotherapists as well as nurses, and indeed anyone interested in reading or writing scholarly articles or research or simply wanting a firm grasp of current research in their field.

Box 10.3   Papers that might be used to start a journal club discussion

- Hemmings A (2000) Counselling in primary care: a review of the practice evidence. *British Journal of Guidance and Counselling* 28:233–52.
- Howey L and Ormrod J (2002) Personality disorder, primary care counselling and therapeutic effectiveness. *Journal of Mental Health* 11:131–9.
- Marwaha S and Johnson S (2005) Views and experiences of employment among people with psychosis: A qualitative descriptive study. *International Journal of Social Psychiatry* 51:302–16.
- Michalak EE, Yatham LN and Lam RW (2005) Quality of life in bipolar disorder: a review of the literature. *BMC Health and Quality of Life Outcomes* 3:72 (www.hqlo.com/content/3/1/72)

A range of question sets has been proposed either to assist generally in critically appraising the literature (*see* Critical Appraisal Skills Programme at www.phru. nhs.uk/casp/casp.htm) or to determine the usefulness for practice. The question sets for usefulness in practice or grading have come in for criticism (Atkins *et al*, 2004). The authors of that critique have gone on to propose their own set of questions for grading the quality of the evidence generated by a study (Grade Working Group, 2004) and begun to evaluate its usefulness (Atkins *et al*, 2005).

Benefits and criticisms of using a systematic approach to reading research

There is evidence (through a systematic review) that postgraduate teaching in evidence-based medicine which included teaching systematic critical appraisal skills did improve knowledge, skills, attitudes and behaviour (Coomarasamy and Khan, 2004). However, the authors were unable to find any studies that evaluated whether such teaching had any direct impact on health outcomes.

How well qualitative research 'fits' into evidence-based practice continues to be debated and explored (Sandelowski, 2004). An earlier assessment of reports of qualitative research in primary care showed that the publications reviewed lacked methodological detail required for adequate critical appraisal (Hoddinott and Pill, 1997). Thus, much of what is published may be useful, but can only be found to be useful if it is carefully scrutinised as described above.

Conclusion

Reading and critically appraising the literature support primary care staff in dealing with patients with a SEMI, by helping each of them identify the current best evidence for practice. Counsellors and psychotherapists reading and critically appraising the literature can only advance the current research climate in their field. It is hoped that this chapter has gone some way in facilitating that process.

References

Agar MH (1997) Ethnography: an overview. *Substance Use and Misuse* 32:1155–73.

Atkins D, Eccles M, Flottorp S et al (2004) Systems for grading the quality of evidence and the strength of recommendations I: Critical appraisal of existing approaches. The GRADE Working Group. *BMC Health Services Research* 4:38. www.biomedcentral.com/1472-6963/4/38 (accessed 15 January 2007).

Atkins D, Briss PA, Eccles M et al (2005) Systems for grading the quality of evidence and the strength of recommendations II: Pilot study of a new system. *BMC Health Services Research* 5:25 www.biomedcentral.com/1472-6963/5/25 (accessed 4 January 2007).

Barnes J, Stein A and Rosenberg W (1999) Evidence-based medicine and evaluation of mental health services: methodological issues and future directions. *Archives of Disease in Childhood* 80:280–5.

Begg C, Cho M, Eastwood S et al (1996) Improving the quality of reporting of randomized controlled trials. The CONSORT statement. *Journal of the American Medical Association* 276:637–9.

Berg A, Fleischer S and Behrens J (2005) Development of two search strategies for literature in MEDLINE-PubMed: nursing diagnoses in the context of evidence-based nursing. *International Journal of Nursing Terminologies and Classifications* 16:26–32.

Boyatzis R (1998) *Transforming Qualitative Information: thematic analysis and code development*. Thousand Oaks: Sage.

Coomarasamy A and Khan KS (2004) What is the evidence that postgraduate teaching in evidence-based medicine changes anything? A systematic review. *British Medical Journal* 329:1017–21.

Cramer JS and Mahoney MC (2001) Introducing evidence-based medicine to the journal club, using a structured pre and post test: a cohort study. *Medical Education* 1:6.

Department of Health (1999) *Clinical Governance in the New NHS*. Health service Circular (HSC 1999/065) www.dh.gov.uk/assetRoot/04/01/20/43/04012043.pdf (accessed 4 January 2007).

Dong P, Wong LL, Ng S, Loh M and Mondry A (2004) Quantitative evaluation of recall and precision of CAT Crawler, a search engine specialised on retrieval of critically appraised topics. *BMC Medical Informatics and Decision Making* 4:21.

Evidence-Based Medicine Working Group (1992) Evidence-based medicine. *Journal of the American Medical Association* 268:2420–5.

Fontelo P, Liu F and Ackerman M (2005) *ask*MEDLINE: a free-text, natural language query tool for MEDLINE/PubMed. *BMC Medical Informatics and Decision Making* 5:5.

Fowkes FGR and Fulton OM (1991) Critical appraisal of published research: introductory guidelines. *British Medical Journal* 302:1136–40.

Glaser B (2002) Conceptualization: on theory and theorizing using grounded theory. *International Journal of Qualitative Methods* 1:Article 3. www.ualberta.ca/~ijqm/ (accessed 4 January 2007).

Grade Working Group (2004) Grading quality of evidence and strength of recommendations. *British Medical Journal* 328:1490. http://bmj.com/cgi/content/full/328/7454/1490 (accessed 4 January 2007).

Greenhalgh T (1997) *How to Read a Paper: the basics of evidence-based medicine*. London: BMJ Publishing Group.

Grimshaw J, McAuley LM, Bero LA *et al* (2003) Systematic reviews of the effectiveness of quality improvement strategies and programmes. *Quality and Safety in Health Care* 12:298–303.

Haynes RB, Wilczynski N, McKibbon KA, Walker CJ and Sinclair JC (1994) Developing optimal search strategies for detecting clinically sound studies in MEDLINE. *Journal of the American Medical Informatics Association* 1:447–58.

Hoddinott P and Pill R (1997) A review of recently published qualitative research in general practice. More methodological questions than answers? *Family Practice* 14:313–19.

Horsburgh D (2002) Evaluation of qualitative research. *Journal of Clinical Nursing* 12:307–12.

Hsieh H and Shannon SE (2005) Qualitative content analysis. *Qualitative Health Research* 15:1277–88.

Jenkins M (2004) Evaluation of methodological search filters – a review. *Health Information and Libraries Journal* 21:148–63.

Jones ML (2004) Application of systematic review methods to qualitative research: practical issues. *Journal of Advanced Nursing* 48:271–8.

Laverty SM (2003) Hermeneutic phenomenology and phenomenology: a comparison of historical and methodological considerations. *International Journal of Qualitative Methods*, 2(3):Article 3. www.ualberta.ca/~iiqm/backissues/2_3final/html/laverty.html (accessed 4 January 2007).

Mays N and Pope C (2000) Qualitative research in health care: assessing quality in qualitative research. *British Medical Journal* 320:50–2.

Meyer J (2000) Qualitative research in health care: using qualitative methods in health related action research. *British Medical Journal* 320:178–81.

Miles M and Huberman A (1994) *Qualitative Data Analysis*.Thousand Oaks: Sage.

Muir Gray JA (1996) *Evidence-based Healthcare: how to make health policy and management decisions*. Oxford: Churchill Livingstone.

Pawson R (2002) Evidence-based policy: the promise of 'realist synthesis'. *Evaluation* 8:340–58.

Pope C, Ziebland S and Mays N (2000) Qualitative research in health care: Analysing qualitative data. *British Medical Journal* 320:114–16.

Rosenberg W and Donald A (1995) Evidence-based medicine: an approach to clinical problem solving. *British Medical Journal* 310:1122–6.

Sandelowski M (2004) Using qualitative research: keynote address to tenth annual Qualitative Health Research Conference. *Qualitative Health Research* 14:1366–86.

Stickley T and Phillips C (2005) Single case study and evidence-based practice. *Journal of Psychiatric and Mental Health Nursing* 12:728–32.

Swift G (2004) How to make journal clubs interesting. *Advances in Psychiatric Treatment* 10:67–72.

Welsh I and Lyons CM (2001) Evidence-based care and the case for intuition and tacit knowledge in clinical assessment and decision making in mental health nursing practice: an empirical contribution to the debate. *Journal of Psychiatric and Mental Health Nursing* 8:299–305.

Whittemore R and Knafl K (2005) The integrative review: updated methodology. *Journal of Advanced Nursing* 52:546–53.

Wilczynski NL and Haynes RB (2006) Optimal search strategies for identifying mental health content in MEDLINE: an analytic survey. *Annals of General Psychiatry* 5:4.

Chapter 11

End piece and last word

John Eatock

Mention 'mental illness' and the word 'mental' often strikes fear into the hearts of the general population of this country. Mention of a person being 'mentally ill', or looking at a referral letter which alludes to a history of mental illness or to a particular condition that has been diagnosed, and many counsellors begin to become exceptionally wary and to also realise that they too are perhaps afraid. Stigma is something that pervades society and it is particularly subversive in the area of mental illness (Carter, 2005). Furthermore, all those working in today's society need to be aware of the contexts of culture, ethnicity and racism with reference to our perception of mental illness. Maurice Lipsedge (Chapter 6) takes us further along the path of understanding that is introduced with a quotation from Jonathan Miller in the chapter by Helen Lester (Chapter 4).

It seems to me that counsellors are afraid because of all the usual factors:

- ignorance and lack of knowledge concerning many diagnosed mental illnesses
- little or no experience of people who are mentally ill beyond the usual tag of 'mild to moderate'
- insufficient training
- a deficiency in understanding the effects of the medication that such people may be receiving.

The immediate response is often that, 'this is beyond my competency', 'this referral needs to go to someone else', 'there is nothing that I can do to help this person', because of what has been written in the notes about a prevailing condition, or one which is under control or from which a person may well be 'in recovery'. Such responses are often entirely reasonable and understandable and can often be correct and appropriate for that particular counsellor at that time. Glyn Hudson-Allez's contribution (Chapter 2) therefore is a timely reminder concerning the issue of assessment and risk for the counsellor, and we know from other studies that this is an area in which all counsellors need to ensure they have adequate training (Hickey, 2005). Furthermore, Glyn gives a clear description of what severe and enduring illnesses look like and what one may expect in working with these individuals. She also points out, not only the importance of good counselling supervision, but the fact that anxiety may exist within the supervisors themselves. The plea for counsellors to extend their range of practice into this area is more than apparent.

Nevertheless, certainly when an individual's condition is 'under control' or they are 'in recovery', there is every possibility that such a client may well benefit from entering into a counselling relationship. A careful reading of the chapter by Robert John Ganderson on living with schizophrenia (Chapter 1) will reveal instances where many people would turn to counsellors for assistance with those, not unusual, events which impinge upon all our lives such as bereavement and loss, the effects of a sudden death, resorting to the abuse of alcohol, being unemployed, maybe issues of trust in relationships and, for the more psychodynamically inclined, living within a family with a history of mental illness. Moreover, having been 'mentally ill' or having been so diagnosed does not exempt any of us from the slings and arrows of everyday life. This being the case, some of those who are referred may well be usefully engaged in counselling and there is a need to be better informed and, if possible, trained in the recognition of mental illness and medication. To this end the British Association of Counselling and Psychotherapy (www.bacp.co.uk) has produced information sheets that are freely available to their members and others at www.bacp.co.uk (Freeth, 2004; Russello, 2005). The need for the exorcism of this fear and stigma is obviously best served by training and experience, and those counsellors who work in the NHS (other than the very few who work in psychiatric departments) are advised to speak to their colleagues, both psychiatrists and others, to rectify this possible deficiency.

Forewarned is also to be forearmed, and Professor Joan Curzio provides us with a very useful overview on how to find evidence on severe and enduring mental illness and how to look at this evidence with a critical eye (Chapter 10). Those of us working in the NHS need to be ever aware of evidence and its usefulness as well as its shortcomings. This chapter is the roadmap of just what counsellors need to know and do in order to get the evidence to advance counselling research.

A knowledge and facility in the use of the 'language of mental health and illness' do not go amiss 'even if one doesn't like it or agree with the concepts of psychiatry' to quote Rachel Freeth, another contributor to this volume (Chapter 7). The use of the framework of the Mental State Examination should not be alien to counsellors who observe their clients in similar, if less formal, ways. The straightforward frameworks that April Russello (Chapter 3) mentions such as the 'three Ps inquiry factors' and the 'four vulnerability factors' could easily be incorporated into a counsellor's practice. Keeping April's chapter on concepts of mental health and illness to hand in the counsellor's room or library would be useful for that day when the 'mentally ill' client walks through the door!

In my own experience in primary care it can be the case that a hard-pressed GP asks that a counsellor 'supports' or offers 'containment' to a patient and indicates that the patient has suffered/is suffering from a mental illness. In this case, although this may be in an exceptional circumstance, to be able to do as asked can be beneficial to that person and reduce the stigma by helping the patient within the primary care team. The general trend in the NHS is away from secondary services wherever possible and towards working collaboratively with colleagues to whom counsellors will be able to offer assistance and their unique contribution to patients who often can feel dehumanised and over-medicalised (Eatock, 2006). Collaborative working and willingness to communicate effectively with colleagues have long been more than desirable qualities for NHS counsellors (Eatock and Russello, 2004), and colleagues such as the general practitioner with a special interest (GPwSI) in mental health can be a valuable resource to a hard-pressed counsellor. The question is, 'Do you know who the GPwSI is?'

The usual problems of everyday life for which counselling may be useful can affect everyone without exception. Indeed Helen Lester (Chapter 4) points out that, for example, for a young person with an FEP, 'it is a life-changing event for the person and their family, all of whom often require long-term support and guidance'. It may be that the counsellor who is a member of the primary care team can make a major contribution to those in whose context mental illness has occurred, namely their family and friends. Richard Byng (Chapter 5) also points out that there is a common impression that 'most common mental health problems are new onset, whereas as many as 60% are recurrent'. The most common of those that a counsellor will see are patients suffering from depression, and this is indeed the meat and drink of the majority of counsellors. Any counsellor casting an eye over the 'three Ds model: inclusion criteria for long-term mental illness' and recalling their own clients will recognise that they have indeed been seeing clients with long-term mental illness. Counselling can, as Richard says, 'be relevant during periods of recovery and a buffer against further relapses'.

The notions of 'counselling support' and 'containment' can give the impression, often common among other health professionals, that this is all that counselling and counsellors do, and so they need to emphasise to their colleagues that counselling is 'the therapeutic use of relationship', demanding considerable skill, and that as such, a referral to the counsellor and a request for their help is more than 'a listening ear' or 'tea and sympathy'. It will in fact be 'therapy'; our educative function with our colleagues is a never-ending task! There is also evidence that those counsellors in both primary and secondary care, despite their fears and hesitations, do in fact see clients who have severe mental health difficulties (Barkham *et al*, 2005). The expansion of 'shared care' means opportunities and challenges that are increasingly available if the counsellor dares to move out of the counselling room and more actively engage with the team that is invariably involved.

Michael Harris's chapter (Chapter 8) provides useful insights into pain as an emotional experience, and should not merely enhance the knowledge and practice of those counsellors working with clients who suffer chronic 'somatic' pain, but should broaden the understanding of many counsellors who have not yet encountered such clients but who may do so in the future. Similarly, Clare Gerada (Chapter 9) reminds counsellors that not only do they see many clients with dual diagnosis, but also that it is highly likely that these clients will have had experience of drug use and that this is likely in that group of people who are frequently referred to their services, namely women with anxiety and depression. That is not the only fact to be gleaned from this chapter which lays bare the situation around co-morbidity and its complexity.

Having said all of the above, the majority of counsellors will be cheered and heartened by the contribution of Rachel Freeth (Chapter 7) on the need for a thorough overhaul of the way that people with psychological and emotional distress are cared for in the NHS. There is little to add except to say that we too share the emancipatory vision of O'Hara (1997) that comes at the end of her chapter. There are hopeful signs as I note the slow but sure advancement of the notion of 'wellbeing' in some NHS documents (National Institute for Mental Health in England, 2005). Notwithstanding the inevitable politics involved, we need to be fully aware ourselves of the politics of this area. All of the above chapters are worthy of being absorbed and worth more than mere consideration, but can be read and read again with something to be gained with every re-reading!

References

Barkham M, Gilbert N, Connell J, Marshall C and Twigg E (2005) Suitability and utility of the CORE-OM and CORE-A for assessing severity of presenting problems in psychological therapy services based in primary and secondary care settings. *British Journal of Psychiatry* 186:239–46.

Carter M (2005) Keep quiet about it. *Community Care* 8–14 December 2005:38–9.

Eatock J (2006) Fitness to be trained: the selection of trainees and course content: a trainer's view. In: Hooper D and Weitz P (eds) *Psychological Therapies in Primary Care: training and training standards*. London: Karnac.

Eatock J and Russello A (2004) The distinctive contribution of counselling/psychotherapy to health and healthcare in Britain. *Healthcare Counselling and Psychotherapy Journal* 4:3.

Freeth R (2004) Information Sheet P8: *Psychopharmacology and Counselling and Psychotherapy*. Rugby: British Association for Counselling and Psychotherapy.

Hickey A (2005) Risk Assessment. *Healthcare Counselling and Psychotherapy Journal* 5:24–7.

National Institute for Mental Health in England (2005) *Making it Possible: improving mental health and well-being in England*. London: Department of Health.

O'Hara M (1997) Emancipatory therapeutic practice in a turbulent transmodern era: a work of retrieval. *Journal of Humanistic Psychology* 37:7–33.

Russello A (2005) Information Sheet G7: Recognising Mental Health and Mental Health Problems. Rugby: British Association for Counselling and Psychotherapy.

Index